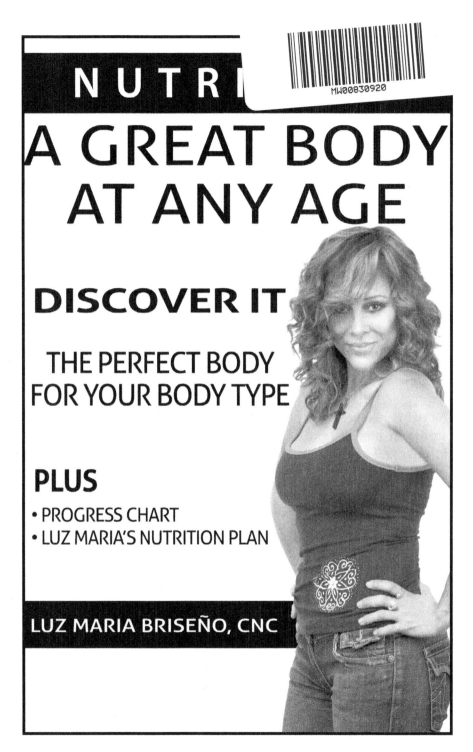

NUTRI

A GREAT BODY AT ANY AGE

DISCOVER IT

THE PERFECT BODY FOR YOUR BODY TYPE

PLUS

- PROGRESS CHART
- LUZ MARIA'S NUTRITION PLAN

LUZ MARIA BRISEÑO, CNC

Cover design: Rodrigo Navarro

Cover picture: David Hadif

Consultant: Armando Villanueva

LUZ MARIA BRISEÑO, CNC

A GREAT BODY AT ANY AGE

ISBN 000-0-000-00000-0

Printed in the United States of America

DEDICATION AND ACKNOWLEDGEMENTS

This book is dedicated to you my faithful listener, who for years has been a part of my show, continually enriching it with a question, a comment, a testimony, a tear. People like you have been my inspiration and an incentive to continue with my mission; the mission of improving your quality of life through nutrition. I thank God for placing so many important people like you in my path.

I thank my son Mateo Bravo, with his birth he gave me the strength to fight against the tide. Armando Villanueva, the man who arrived so unexpectedly in my life and turned it completely around the way it happens only in Hollywood movies. To my best friend Dr. Eduardo Lopez Navarro, the most amazing human being that I have ever met; his friendship and advice have helped me grow in all aspects of my life.

DISCLAIMER

This book does not, in any way, shape or form reflect the views of my employer Univision Radio or any of its employees; its sole objective is to provide nutritional information that I have learned in the alternative search for good health. The information contained herein is not intended to replace medical recommendations or treatments.

The nutrition plan that I recommend in this book is the one that I utilize every day with excellent results. I, Luz María Briseño, certified nutrition consultant CNC, am not responsible for any allergic reaction that you may result from the consumption of any of the recommended foods in this book.

Keep in mind that each person's body is different; what has worked for me may not necessarily work for you. If any food or vitamin causes an allergic reaction or makes you ill, stop using it and call your doctor or go to a nearby hospital immediately. Consult with a physician prior to following any recommendations made on this book.

WHAT IS NUTRITION?

The definition of nutrition in its vast meaning... is the process or a series of processes in which live organisms in their complete form or each of its components, parts or organs maintain themselves in their normal living and growing condition. The word nutrition is also defined as the provision of the necessary materials in the form of sustenance to maintain cells and organisms with life. Many common health problems can be prevented or healed with good nutrition. Nutrition is the study of the relationship between foods and drinks to health or illnesses.

Nutrition is a form of helping the body with the tools to better illnesses without the use of toxic drugs. It is basically like giving the body the tools to do what it can naturally achieve on its own... to heal itself. Nutrition will not cover up the problem, nor will it treat its symptoms of illness, it will in turn repair the body's damage from the root. Multiple health problems will better themselves simultaneously and degenerative illnesses will be prevented.

Being that each person has a different structure type, to achieve an optimal nutrition we must learn to listen to our body's necessities and focus on maintaining it healthy in its totality, not by only healing that part of the body that is not functioning adequately; as each person has a different physical chemistry, one that is unique due to the its environment and genetics, we also have to recognize our own metabolism type. Nutrition is not a diet, but a lifestyle that will keep you vital; the speed, effectiveness and way in which this will work is dependent on how many health problems you may have, how long you may have had these, your age, your genetics, your lifestyle and your desire to make true changes to reach a firm discipline... to love your body and start taking care of it.

Generally, the first changes are achieved in 3 days, sometimes it can take 2 weeks, and in other cases up to 6 weeks or even months being that it will require time to repair the intestinal flora, cleanse the body of internal garbage and nurture each cell. The body's cells will regenerate themselves about every 6 weeks; we must have patience being that the symptoms took months or even decades in their formation due to your lifestyle. With nutrition recovery is not instant but if you persevere and take care of your body, you will find incredible results. Remember that for every 12 months that you abused your body or simply didn't nurture it, now you will need to eat healthy for 6 weeks. With this in consideration, take paper and pencil or a calculator... time to calculate. Remember that for each year of bad eating you will need 6 weeks of good nutrition.

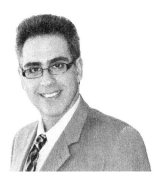

Dr. Eduardo López Navarro

Informative, detailed, practical, complete and extremely motivating. All of these and many more adjectives describe Luz María Briseño's new book, nutritionist by excellence and host of a radio program. With regards to nutrition this book is a work of art, one which clearly, precisely, and directly promotes nutrition at all intensities and colors. You have in your hands a complete encyclopedia to be able to live a sane and healthy life through nutrition. Through the extensive content of this treasure you will discover that great body that now sleeps within you, waiting to awaken. Upon reading it I know that your first reaction will be to express in a loud voice the same words that I called out... with great respect words I took from her majesty... "YEAH BABY!"

TABLE OF CONTENTS

A GREAT BODY AT ANY AGE
THE FUNDAMENTAL BASICS OF NUTRITION

- The secret of burning fat as a fuel

- Tea that will strengthen the immunological system (Immune Tea)

- An explanation of its use

- An explanation of its use

INTRODUCTION

Suffering almost always makes us want to change, but having this suffering always present also helps us never abandon change. This is why we must always remember that suffering is the last tool we have to make a change... because if this suffering doesn't make us change, like Dr. Eduardo López Navarro always says... nothing will.

Many people mature with age and others need to suffer to do something for ourselves. If age and this suffering are not enough to change a sedentary lifestyle, the effects of obesity, diabetes, cardiovascular diseases, depression and other health problems will end your health and by logical consequence with your happiness and desire to live. A balanced diet has always been the base of good health because our body has the power of self-healing. This is why you need the necessary tools: protein, carbohydrates, quality fats, vitamins, minerals, exercise, rest and water, plenty of water.

What causes most illnesses? It is said that a high percentage of illnesses are genetically caused; a number that increases due to a sedentary lifestyle. Other theories ensure that over 80% of illnesses are caused by chronic stress. If you add the lack of exercise, the excess of junk food consumed, adding the chemicals with which the body is being nurtured and you don't drink water; your genetics and lifestyle will debilitate your defense system. The weaker your immunological system is, the least amount of antibodies will be available to fight against the free radicals, viruses, bacteria and toxins that daily are attacking your body.

"A Great Body At Any Age" is designed to help you, being that you are tired of suffering due to any illness caused by having a bad nutrition, due to the abuse of synthetic foods. This book will motivate you and to have you better your health so that you can prevent degenerative illnesses through nutrition by implementing a new lifestyle. If you are of the people that say not to have time to exercise, but do find the time to smoke, drink alcohol, frequently use medication, not eat healthy, work too hard, not sleep your 8 hours, and have health and emotional problems and to top it off junk food is your primary source of nutrition... How long do you think your body will resist? Maybe when you find yourself in an emergency room you will then "have time" to think and reconsider the importance of "making time for yourself"; time to plan what you will eat during the day and to exercise.

What is the most important appointment on your itinerary? The appointment with yourself... With this, not only will you feel better physically, mentally and emotionally, but will set an example for the people that love and admire you... your loved ones.

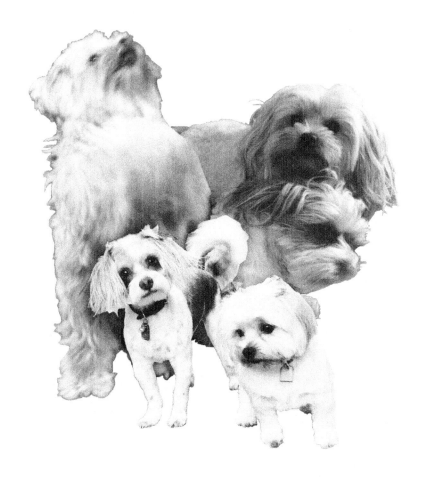

A GREAT BODY AT ANY AGE

THE BASIC FOUNDATION OF NUTRITION

FATTY ACIDS VERSUS MUSCLES

Fatty acids and essential oils represent the same; they are a chain of molecules that form part of a natural fat that the body needs to appropriately function, of which can be found in natural oils and non-saturated fats; these are said to be essential as they are not produced by the body, they are needed for its function.

Nerve cells and brain tissue are insulated with fat as if they were electric cables. Each of the membranes surrounding each cell needs fatty acids (essential oils) to control the entry and exit of materials. Cholesterol is indispensable for hormonal function including sexual and adrenal glands; it is also one of the fats that forms the body's cell membranes. Essential oils are the body's lubricant, necessary for the proper function of the brain, heart, liver, eyes, skin and digestive system.

THE FUNCTION OF FAT CELLS

Fat cells are in charge of producing fat with sugars and fatty acids, those which release energy to help the rest of the cells to function properly. When the fat cells receive emergency signals they immediately start to work and start to store fat that will later be converted and used as energy. Being that these fat cells grow in size they will need more space and logically if they don't have this space, they will create it; this way creating new cells that will later be filled with fat.

FAT... BURNS FAT

When you eat only once a day or deprive yourself of eating for many hours, cells receive a false signal of emergency and immediately the body takes intelligent and drastic action: they store fat to later be used in critical moments of hunger. This is why we need to eat 5 to 6 times a day and include essential oils.

At an older age, additional fatty cells substitute the muscle cells and being that the muscles require more energy to function, once the muscle cells are replaced by fatty cells the body no longer needs substituted energy, instead it will need fatty acids to metabolize the excess fat. As we age, this is why our metabolism slows down and the body needs less food, but it does need food with a higher nutrition value.

- So that you can see the benefits of exercise it should be done in a 20 minute workout period or more and consume essential oils after every meal. Interrupted movement allows for the heart to pump at a faster pace, providing the body with large quantities of oxygen that allow the body to burn fat, but this will not happen in the absence of lubricating fatty acids. The exercises that will produce this effect are jogging, jump roping, bicycling, and walking at a fast pace.

- Consistency is more important than the intensity of the exercise being performed. Exercise and essential oils help develop muscle; while the fat is used as energy that allows for muscle growth.

- When stimulants are used (weight loss pills) without a good nutrition, they body's chemistry changes and muscle tissue is lost; when you stop taking these stimulants or metabolism stimulants, weight gain is once again present, and sometimes up to twice the weight because the body's chemistry registers the body chemistry of an obese person, and you will not recover the lost muscle.

• The fat in your food has a chemical composition similar to the one of your body; this is why it can store it with such ease. If the fat is consumed in moderate quantities along with essential oils like Omega3, it is digested with ease. This is why the body does not recognize hydrogenated foods or low fat foods. These are not metabolized as they are not identified.

DEFICIENCY OF FATTY ACIDS AND RELATED PROBLEMS

Health problems related with essential oil deficiencies: dry skin and hair, premature wrinkles, congested liver, gastrointestinal problems, memory loss, cardiovascular problems, allergies, candidiasis, acne, psoriasis, eczema and other types of skin infections (body, hands, feet and scalp).

FOODS HIGH IN ESSENTIAL FATTY ACIDS

There are 2 categories of essential oils: Omeg3 and Omega6.

Omega3 consists of: alpha-linolenic acid and eicosapentaenoic acid (EPA); these are found in foods such as: fish and fish oils, flaxseed and walnut.

Omega6 consists of: linoleic acid and gamma-linolenic acid that are found in such foods: raw nuts, legumes, pumpkin seeds, sesame seeds, sunflower seeds, etc.... and in some vegetable oils like evening primrose oil, vitamin E, grape seed oil, soy bean oil, olive oils, sesame oil, green-leaf vegetables and borage oil.

To obtain the benefits of Omega3 and Omega6 they must be consumed in their raw form. Heat or the use of these to prepare foods will reduce the nutrition value and even worse, free radicals are formed that are toxic and poisonous.

ESSENTIAL OILS IN THE FORM OF SUPPLEMENTS

To better any health condition related with low levels of fatty acids, make sure to keep a balanced diet, a moderate consumption of sugars. Avoid processed foods, refined and high in saturated fat. Consume essential oils through the foods you eat and if at all possible in form of a supplement. Drink plenty of water, exercise and meditate.

If you are a woman above the age of 18 and suffer with a skin condition, hormonal changes, cardiovascular and respiratory irregularities, you can take 1300 mg of primrose oil once a day. The maximum dosage is 1300 mg twice a day in severe cases, severe or chronic.

If you are a man with hormonal, skin or cardiovascular problems, avoid primrose oil. You may consume essential oils in form of fish oil; you can take Omega3, (two capsules after each meal is what is recommended). Omega3 can be consumed by both men and women, but not the evening primrose oil, this is only for women.

If a man was to take this, there will be a hormonal change reaction that will make him more emotional and sensitive.

NOTE: Women with breast cancer related with a unbalance of estrogen, avoid primrose oil. Consider taking Black currant seed oil.

WATER

Being thirsty is a sign that our organism is dehydrated. When we sweat a lot or when we get sick of diarrhea or insolation or fever or we suffer of sunburn or we drink antibiotics, and on top of this we eat junk food, our body's fluids get so low that there is no other option than to steal water from our saliva. If you are the type of person that will not drink water even if you are thirsty, it will not take long for you to feel the effect of dehydration and with this fatigue, irritability, headaches, and general discomfort. Do not wait too long to drink water.

Liquids such as water, milk, juice and tea should be consumed in between meals so that you don't drown the digestive enzymes. This is why you should only drink from 4 to 6 ounces of water, juice or milk after every meal. Preferably, wait 15 minutes after you are done eating to drink any type of liquid. Each time you drink water in between meals, be sure to drink approximately 8 ounces at a time so that you don't get too full; but if after drinking the 8 ounces of water you are still feeling thirsty and hungrier than normal, you are going to urinate with more frequency, your skin, your lips and mouth are dry and you feel extremely fatigued, you will have to go to the doctor.

Being that water is approximately 60% of our organism, it is a primary component of our body. Drinking water helps maintain our blood levels in their place, the lymphatic system will keep itself clean and circulating properly, the digestive system will produce its gastric juices, the body's temperature and formation of tears will be regulated. Urine and sweat will also be maintained at their appropriate levels.

It is important to say that the circulatory system, the skeletal system, the nervous system, the immune system and the digestive system will be affected with the lack of water. Water carries electrolytes; these are salt minerals that help transport the body's electrical currents. The principal salt minerals are: sodium, potassium, calcium, magnesium and chloride.

HOW MUCH WATER SHOULD WE DRINK?

The body's requirements for water for each person will vary and have to do with corporal weight, lifestyle, nutrition, exercise and even weather. To know what the required quantity of water for the body's proper function, you will need to divide half of what you weigh in pounds, by 8. Your result will be the total quantity of 8 ounce cups of water that you must drink throughout the day. On hotter days you must drink 2 additional cups; when you do physical exercise, you will then have to drink 2 additional 8 ounce cups of water. As an example, the "big eared" as I call my assistant Alex Russo, weighs 220 pounds, half would be 110 pounds, divided by 8, would equal 13.75 cups of 8 ounces of water.

NOTE: Even if Alex should be drinking 14 cups of water, it is not recommended. The maximum that any person should drink is 12 cups of water or the equivalent of 3 liters of water per day.

WARNING ON DRINKING MORE THAN 3 LITERS OF WATER

Drinking more than 3 liters of water a day causes health problems due to the excessive loss of minerals. Drinking more than 5 liters of water a day can cause hyponatremia or intoxication; intoxication occurs when the regular levels of the body's sodium are lowered with the excess of water being that it dilutes the sodium from the blood stream and causes edema, cerebral inflammation. Symptoms: nausea, vomiting, convulsions, weakness, coma and death.

IS THERE A RISK TO DRINKING FAUCET WATER?

Every city is different and there is no sufficient proof showing how detrimental faucet water can be, it would be best to avoid the risk. In some cities faucet water has high levels of sodium; this is relevant to cardiovascular problems like high blood pressure.

When these high levels of sodium biologically replace such important body minerals as calcium and magnesium, the resistance of the body is affected that prevent heart attacks or illnesses.

Faucet water in most cities of this country have a high level of chlorine, these used to kill germs; too much fluoride to prevent dental problems and even alkaline substances to change the acid or PH in the water. Although the alkaline substances are used to prevent corrosion of the pipes of faucet water, there is no guarantee of the presence of toxic metals like esbirro, lead, mercury, aluminum and cadmium.

A major problem is that all of these synthetic substances that are used to bring faucet water can be carcinogens.

PURIFIED WATER

Most faucet water comes from the surface of reserves formed from rivers, lakes, or other subterranean reserves. This water goes through local plants for purification and filtration using sand, gravel and chemicals that help convert contaminated water into fit to drink water for humans.

THE BEST BOTTLED WATER

One of the best bottled waters is known as "spring water", this water is obtained from subterranean lands and is treated with chlorine but it is not processed, this is why its taste is different and even conserves its natural minerals.

HOW HEALTHY IS SPARKLING WATER?

All water is "mineral", but the bottled mineral water known as "sparkling water", along with carbon dioxide (CO2), contains many more minerals than the rest. "Seltzer" is carbonated water with carbon dioxide, bottled mineral waters contain this. "Club Soda" is basically the same, except that this has more minerals than the rest.

The question is, how healthy is it to drink commercial mineral water? I think that it is enough to know that carbon dioxide (CO2) is a colorless, odorless, flavorless gas that is soluble in water. This gas extracts oxygen 150% stronger than the air your breath from your organism. We find carbon dioxide in nature. Plants convert carbon dioxide into oxygen just as you and I convert carbon dioxide into oxygen when we exhale, we exhale carbon dioxide.

Carbon dioxide is used not only in carbonated drinks or minerals, but also in dry snow and fire extinguishers. Indeed, it is dangerous to abuse drinking mineral water because it will rob you of the oxygen in the cells of your body and brain, and we need oxygen to live. In other words, carbon dioxide or Seltzer (water with carbon dioxide that bubbles when there is no pressure) will asphyxiate brain cells because it will rob its oxygen; therefore causing headaches, dizziness, and loss of concentration.

WATER PURIFIERS

Filtered water is simply the result of the extraction or removal of up to 99.75% of chemicals, metals and bacteria. There are about 2 million purification systems from which to choose from. Many experts agree that the two best water purifiers for the home are a double ozone filter and the reverse osmosis purifier; the double ozone filter is not easy to find and its price may not be too accessible for low income families. On the other hand, multi-carbon filter systems and reverse osmosis purifiers have two or more purification mechanisms that remove almost 100% of organic materials. This water purification system is available in different sizes, from units for the home to industrial size units. These purifiers used to be costly, but recently can be found at economic and competitive prices. These can be easily found and purchased through internet websites.

DISTILLED WATER

Distilled water is not recommended for daily use being that it does not have any type of minerals. Also, the distilling process requires vaporization at high temperatures. Heating water at 212 degrees Fahrenheit will change the natural chemistry of the water; drinking this will have a biochemical effect in the body that will also be different.

Distilled water is recommended only when it is required to purify the organism. Distilled water easily removes toxins and the excess of minerals from the body.

Plants, tea, vegetables and foods will release more properties and minerals if they are boiled or cooked with distilled water.

REASONS TO DRINK WATER

If you drink water you will feel lighter and full of energy, you will reach your ideal weight, you will get sick less often and if you do get sick you will recuperate much faster. Your kidneys will function better and with this you will prevent severe intoxications, your digestive system will function better and your skin will look younger and fresh.

SUMMARY

Being that we all need water to survive, the best way to drink it is through a purification system that filters toxic substances for the body and also one that does not destroy all minerals. Solid carbon filters do an excellent job in removing chemicals from the water. Reverse osmosis filters even at a higher price than the solid carbon filter also remove almost 100% of the chemicals, bacteria, nitrites and the excess of fluoride from the water without damaging its natural minerals; these purifiers are easy to install and are made of stainless steel.

When you go on vacation you run the risk of infections due to bacteria, parasites, metals, chemicals or radioactivity found in the water. It would be best to take your own water, but if your trip is

long and taking enough water is not possible, then at least be sure that you boil the water at least 10 minutes before drinking it. Boiling water for 1 minute will destroy bacteria and parasites, boiling water for 10 minutes will destroy viruses found in the water. Even though you are assuring yourself that you are drinking multi minerals, only in a case of emergency you are allowed to add 10 drops of iodine for every liter of water and let it rest for 30 minutes prior to its use, this will destroy the germs.

CRAVINGS

EMOTIONAL CRAVINGS

The popular "cravings" for sugary foods are generally psychologically caused due to boredom, anxiety, habit, or just because this is what you eat. You must resist for at least 5 to 10 minutes, this is the approximate time that a craving lasts until it passes over. Cravings sometimes get misinterpreted with hunger, but in reality what you may be is thirsty... you just may be thirsty. Stress caused by emotional problems is the general cause of cravings for sugary foods, especially chocolate. Sugary foods as well as chocolate stimulate the brain which in turn releases endorphin (a brain neurotransmitter that relieves pain) and dopamine (a brain neurotransmitter that produces the sensation of well-being). When you have low levels of serotonin (another neurotransmitter of the central nervous system that wears down with emotional stress), dopamine and endorphin, you will generally also have anxiety attacks, depression and cravings for carbohydrates and sugary foods. Changing your eating habits will allow for the levels of these chemicals to regulate.

If your anxiety for eating sugary foods is related with emotional stress (remember that these anxiety attacks only last 10 minutes), take these minutes of anxiety to analyze yourself; investigate in your subconscious and find out where this anxiety and stress is coming from. This will help you distract your mind for these 10 minutes and at the same time it will also help you confront your emotions. The best techniques to reduce your levels of stress are to practice yoga, do exercise, swim or any other type of physical exercise of choice.

CRAVINGS VERSUS GLUCOSE IMBALANCES

If you are accustomed to eat foods with no nutritional value and are constantly suffering of cravings, it is very probable that your last meal had too many refined carbohydrates; or simply a fact that your body hungers for nutrients. That is to say, when you eat high volumes of refined carbohydrates, your sugar level elevates and your pancreas will begin to release insulin. When the insulin level is high, the sugar level lowers, and when your sugar level is low, your body gets desperate and wishes to obtain an immediate dose of sugar like the one that is found in refined sugary foods and fast food.

This is why your brain sends signals of hunger through anxiety for sugary foods. To avoid these lows or glucose shocks, MAKE SURE that you have a nutritious breakfast and that it is not donuts with coffee. During the day eat nutritious snacks that have protein and fiber so that you can avoid these anxiety attacks or cravings for sugary foods.

You may have noticed that in the mornings you are not all that hungry; take advantage of this balance so that you may eat something of nutritional value, because after this first healthy meal it will be difficult for you to have these glucose shocks, hence you will not have the anxiety for sugary foods. Once you begin your day with white flours or refined sugary foods, it will be very difficult to control your cravings for sugary foods the rest of the day, not even with strong willpower.

CRAVINGS AND STRESS

If your nourishment is balanced, but not necessarily perfect, and you exercise regularly and drink enough water and are still

suffering of anxiety attacks and have cravings for sugary foods, it is almost certain that you are deficient of vitamins and minerals; even if you are taking vitamins it is possible that your body is not absorbing them due to an excess of stress. The next time that you feel with the irrepressible desire to eat some chips or cookies with soda, interrupt this craving by doing something that will keep your mind completely busy, drink 8 ounces of water, eat a fruit (apple) with almonds, or go exercise, remember that this craving will only last 10 minutes.

NOTE: Be careful not to replace one craving with another, like going shopping, smoking or drinking alcohol, because it is very common to replace a bad habit with another, or a negative emotion with another.

CRAVINGS ASSOCIATED WITH NICOTINE

A theory exists that people that smoke will have stronger cravings for sugary foods, suffer of depression, anxiety, and will have psychological problems compared to people that don't smoke. At the same time it is said that the nicotine found in cigarettes will stimulate the false sensation of well-being to be able to deal with anxiety problems and depression. Cigarettes are related to illnesseslike schizophrenia, bipolar disorder, hyperactivity, depression, manic, memory loss and can also be related to the use of drugs and alcohol. People that smoke daily are considered to have a 174% higher risk of suicide compared to people that smoke occasionally. Some private companies and on occasions public companies are utilizing this information to justify the non-hiring of compulsive smokers.

NIGHT CRAVINGS

Generally it is at night when it is more difficult to deal with the famous cravings for sugary foods; the reason why this comes to be is because throughout the day, your diet is in need of more protein and complex carbohydrates, essential oils and less refined sugars or processed foods. If to the previously mentioned you were to add 2 fruits a day it would be much better. Avoid snacks with carbohydrates at night time; this is to avoid having you go to bed with high levels of insulin, avoiding you to burn fat when sleeping. A protein snack is best to have at night; the exception to this would be to have protein from milk, unless it is unsweetened almond milk. Another reason why cravings may attack at night is because cravings are closely related to habits and if one of these habits is watching television while you eat, now that your are concerned with your weight gain it may be concerning to have these cravings at night when you are settling in and watching television. What you can do in this case is to understand that this is only a habit and that your body does not really need this snack you are craving, drink water or have a protein snack or even change your usual activity for 10 days, instead of watching television, read a book or do something different; remember that any activity that you repeat for 10 days straight will be habit forming.

NUTRITIONAL SNACKS TO CALM YOUR DEMONS

If you enjoy sweet bread, chips, or any other type of candy or snack, don't have these in your house; these can be a great temptation at a moment of anxiety. Snacks that you can have are: Almonds, fruit, raw pumpkin or sunflower seeds, natural yogurt or cottage cheese with fruit, yogurt smoothies with skim milk and frozen fruit, wraps prepared with fresh turkey ham and avocado, turkey with tomato and avocado wrapped in a lettuce leaf, if you want to use a tortilla,

be sure to use a tortilla made with sprouted grain. You can drink a skim milk smoothie with a small delicious apple or a slice of toasted sprouted grain bread with a slice of eggplant previously roasted and topped with tomato prepared the following way: dice onion and garlic and cook them on a Teflon pan, add the diced tomato when the onion is roasted and add sea salt, a pinch of pepper and oregano.

When everything is cooked, move the pan away from the stove and add a spoonful of olive oil and a few lemon drops. Lastly, over the toasted bread with the slice of eggplant and tomato, you can add a little grated soy roasted cheese. In addition to this, to a slice of toast you can add avocado, cheese and the following salsa that will require the following food processor preparation: add half of a bunch of parsley, ½ of an onion, 2 medium-sized tomatoes, ½ of a bell pepper, 4 garlic cloves, juice from a medium sized lemon, sea salt and 2 spoonful's of olive oil.

If you would like, you can add 1 or 2 fresh jalapeños (not in vinegar). Lastly, remember that due to the fiber found in apples, they will give you the sensation of being full and because of their natural sugar, they will immediately elevate your mood... they are also not fattening and have vitamins and minerals.

REPLACE SIMPLE CARBOHYDRATES FOR COMPLEX ONES

Replace simple sugars or refined carbohydrates for complex carbohydrates. These will gradually free sugars, this way avoiding glucose lows or shocks and at the same time anxiety attacks. Complex carbohydrates are whole grain foods, including sprouted grains and vegetables.

Avoid eating carbohydrates by themselves; to maintain glucose levels in their place it is best if you eat carbohydrates with protein and essential oils. For example, fish or chicken with vegetables and a salad with olive oil or a single fruit with cheese.

Be careful with the excess of salt, this will release the craving for sugary foods. If you are susceptible to refined sugars, it is best not to have them. Many people can eat a dessert and stop, on the other hand other people in addition to sugary foods; they cannot control themselves once they have eaten sugar... this is why I don't recommend having them.

If day to day at around 11:00 AM you feel the anxiety to have a cream filled glaze donut, a bagel with cream cheese or sweet bread with coffee, this means that you are in need of a more substantial breakfast with fiber or protein. If you stopped eating red meat but you have a craving for it and don't have a balanced diet, one that doesn't include beans or green veggies, it is likely that you are in need of iron, especially if you have chipped fingernails and split ends on your hair.

IMPORTANT: Remember, if you have cravings because you are truly hungry, choose nutritious snacks that will calm your appetite and anxiety, but if you have cravings due to emotional problems, it is only a period of 10 minutes that you must control the craving, but more important, you must find help to heal any emotional wound that needs resolving.

SUPPLEMENTS FOR ANXIETY

These supplements along with a better nutrition and exercise will help place your organism in balance more rapidly. If in 6 weeks you don't see a notable improvement with your emotional cravings, you may have to get psychological help.

Greens (green vegetables in a powder form): Instead of a dose twice a day, take a dose four times a day; each dose with 8 ounces of water with lemon, no sugar.

- Multivitamins with minerals: 1 with breakfast and 1 with lunch

- 500 mg of Vitamin B5 Panthotenic Acid

- Omega3 (Essential Fatty Acids) follow the indications on the bottle

- 3000 mgs of Vitamin C

- 1 capsule for your adrenal glands 3 times a day

- 10 cups with 8 ounces of water a day

- 500 mg of L-Glutamine 2 times a day before breakfast and lunch (only for people over 18 years of age that are not lactating or pregnant)

- 400 Units of Vitamin E

- Liquid calcium citrate 1 ounce on an empty stomach once a day

SUGARS

THE SAD AND SOUR REALITY OF SUGAR

With all the sweetness found in white sugar, corn syrup, maple syrup and raw sugar... reality is really sour. Raw sugar known as brown sugar has more molasses; molasses is the honey of refined brown sugar. When you eat any type of sugar it goes directly to the blood, then to the brain, this is not digested. This causes chemical and hormonal imbalances that later provoke many physical and emotional illnesses.

PROBLEMS RELATED WITH THE ABUSE OF SUGARS

Any type of refined sugar causes an increase in appetite even after we are done eating; it takes the calcium, proteins and nutrients from our food. It provokes hyperactivity in children and adults, it causes headaches, it slows down children's learning process, and it feeds cancerous cells. It changes the chemistry in the brain, it unmeasurably burns cerebral hormones, it coagulates the blood, it concentrates cholesterol, and it decontrols the hormones in the pancreas and insulin and will cause an increase in the size of your liver and kidneys, causing these to work inadequately as these grow in size.

Refined sugars are also the cause of the formation of kidney stones, the excess of acids in the stomach, ulcers, intestinal cancer, it attacks and debilitates the immunological, the skeletal, circulatory, respiratory and nervous systems. The excess of sugar deposits fats in the blood, it interferes with the digestive system – it provokes diarrhea or constipation, varicose veins, cellulitis, hemorrhoids, allergies, it weakens the teeth and worst of all, sugar is like a drug, it is addictive.

The best way to enjoy sweet foods is in its natural form, like fruit or utilizing a natural sweetener like the leaf of the stevia plant. Stevia is a Paraguay native plant that in addition to providing its sweet taste, 0 calories and fiber, this fiber protects the friendly bacteria found in the intestines (lactobacillus and bifid bacteria).

Friendly bacteria keep the intestinal flora in good shape; this way improving intestinal movement, it helps fortify the immunological system, it helps control the formation of free radicals, it keeps the colon clean and it helps the livers performance.

The sweetener stevia can be used to make smoothies, malts, tea, lemonade, etc. This sweetener can be used by persons that suffer from diabetes and can be found in stores and nutrition centers; this can also be found at a more economical price online.

IMPORTANT: Know that for every ¼ spoonful of sugar you eat, the immunological system will slow down or weaken for up to 3 hours. During these 3 hours the body will be more vulnerable and it will be much easier for it to catch a virus or bacteria, especially if someone close suffers from influenza or any contagious illness.

LOSE WEIGHT FOR LIFE

THE EASIEST WAY TO LOSE WEIGHT

AVOID not eating on schedule as much as possible. Avoid eating white flours and refined sugars like cakes, donuts, nachos, chips, cookies, chocolates, coffee, soft drinks, sports drinks, alcohol, cigarettes and fried food. All of this is poison for your body, and if you don't avoid this poison you will not lose weight and won't better your health (if you eat a dessert, only eat it once in a while, and most important... eat it in small quantities).

AVOID gluten; gluten is a protein – a carbohydrate that is found in most grains such as wheat, rye and barley; replace these with bean sprout, these do not have flour or gluten and can be found in most nutrition stores or supermarkets where they specialize in organic foods.

INCLUDE with your food brown rice, millet, and buckwheat, beans of all types, lentil and legumes (vegetables that grow on vines). Chicken breast, white fish, turkey and salmon are some of the animal proteins that you can eat moderately (be sure that these are chewed properly) in small portions, grilled, in its own juice, in the oven or steamed (nothing fried).

DON'T FORGET that the digestive enzymes that you get from eating raw vegetables and in salads with lemon, olive oil and sea salt; these help you have a better digestion and help you absorb nutrients and being that they are high in natural fiber, they act like a mop and broom for your intestines; this way avoiding constipation and logically will help you lose weight faster. If you are malnourished, you will gain the necessary weight and it will better your health.

DO SOME EXERCISE and be sure to break a sweat (a total of 120 minutes per week). Breaking a sweat by doing exercise 4 times a week for at least 30 minutes at a time you will achieve the basic exercise to avoid illnesses and avoid obesity; of course, this type of minimal exercise works only if you combine this with a balanced diet.

DRINK WATER and stop living in a state of dehydration. You need to drink approximately 2.5 liters of water a day. If you suffer of obesity, divide half of your weight by 8; the result will determine the quantity of 8 ounce cups of water you must drink per day. Oh...! When it gets hot, you will need to add two extra cups, and if you exercise... an additional two.

EAT 5 OR 6 TIMES PER DAY making sure to eat 15 to 20 grams of protein (chicken, fish, egg whites, plain yogurt and legumes 4 times a day), but don't try to eat gigantic portions each of these 5 or 6 times, no. You must eat small portions every 3 hours so that your metabolism maintains active and burns any extra fat in your body.

DON'T SKIP BREAKFAST. Breakfast is indispensable if you wish to lose weight, nurture yourself or better your health. This prevents sudden hunger attacks at night and at the same time it will ignite your metabolism. Not because it is important to eat breakfast means that you will eat like it is normally done in the United States. One of the favorite breakfasts in America: A stack of pancakes, 3 scrambled eggs, fried potatoes, bacon, toast, and even a malt; no, this will poison your liver.

It is best to eat something light but nutritious like natural yogurt with fruit, a scrambled egg with vegetables and a slice of sprouted grain bread for breakfast. You can also eat natural oatmeal with fruit or a cup of flourless cereal or gluten with soy milk and almonds.

This kind of light breakfast won't interfere with the livers detoxification. Your liver is always cleaning your organism all through the night and morning, it must eliminate all toxins, but if you eat a gigantic breakfast instead of eliminating toxins, the liver will quit this job and will work on metabolizing the big breakfast (fat) you just ate.

DO NOT FORGET TO CARRY SNACKS TO YOUR CAR AND TAKE THEM TO WORK... always have these with you. You can have almonds, pumpkin seeds, sliced fruit, sliced vegetables, soy cheese and sprouted bread toast. It is best to have a snack than to have an empty stomach.

NOTE: Most important for weight loss is to **eat small portions of food** every 3 hours to maintain your metabolic system working, **drink water** to get rid of toxins that acidify the organism and will not let you lose weight, and **do exercise** to lower your stress levels that are also the reason for being overweight and obese.

DISCIPLINE AND GOOD HABITS

1. Drink plenty of water; divide half of your weight by 8 and the result is the total of 8 ounce cups of water that you must drink during the day, especially between meals.

2. Don't drink water when you are eating; you must drink liquids 15 minutes before or after you eat.

3. Prepare smaller portions of food, properly chew your food and avoid eating when you are upset. Eating while in a negative

emotional state will cause intestinal spasms and a bad absorption.

4. Eat 2 fruits, 2 salads, and 2 portions of vegetables every day, fruits are recommended between meals as well as raw vegetable or semi-raw. If you have never eaten raw cruciferous vegetables (cabbage, broccoli, cauliflower, and Brussel sprouts), start by eating these steamed and gradually semi-cooked, until you can tolerate eating these raw. This type of vegetable tends to cause intestinal inflammation if you don't have enough digestive enzymes.

5. Gradually eliminate fried foods, processed, with chemicals, white flours, refined sugars, and all types of carbonated drinks. Making gradual changes will help you make these permanent and life-lasting.

6. Eat your three main meals and two snacks in between meals at the same schedule time every day; do not let 3 hours go by without eating. So that you are hungry every 3 hours, you must eat small portions of food... logically.

7. Do not eliminate rice, bread, or whole grain foods from your diet; it is a lie that these will make you gain weight; these will avoid having anxiety attacks and cravings to eat flours and refined sugars, these will also give you energy and are the mop and broom of your intestines. The best carbohydrates are the complex ones, these are vegetables and germinated whole grains (if you are not allergic to gluten that is found in wheat, you can go ahead and eat bread, tortillas and cereal made from wheat, but if you suffer of any serious illness, avoid gluten).

8. Do not eat too much of a single food, no matter how healthy it is, this will release allergic reactions to certain foods.

9. Do not eat great quantities of any type of meat, especially if it is fried. Fried meat lasts up to 48 hours to digest. While your small intestine is trying to digest this meat, your stomach will remain jammed, filled with the rest

of the food that you are eating. This will cause indigestion, bad absorption of nutrients and the purification of foods that will eventually convert into bacteria and grave illnesses.

10. Eat a little of everything, but don't remain hungry or too full. When you do sin by eating dessert or something not too healthy, make sure that it is a small portion. If you do commit this sin, enjoy it and don't feel guilty. Guilt acidifies your organism and holds up digestion. If you are sick, it is best to avoid these temptations. If you are compulsive and won't hold back with desserts, don't even taste them. It is best to just eat a fruit.

11. Drink dark green vegetable smoothies (use a blender) with carrots, beets, celery roots, and parsley along with its leaves (8 ounces with breakfast and 8 ounces with lunch), these will purify the blood stream, will calm hunger and the craving or anxiety for sugary foods; these will nurture you and help you lose weight (if you suffer of obesity), but if you're underfed, eating these will help you gain weight.

12. Eat mixed milled seeds: flaxseed, chia, sunflower, sesame, and pumpkin seed. These are an excellent source of essential oils and fiber. These will not only help you rejuvenate, but will also help prevent digestive system and colon illnesses.

13. Drink a spoonful of wheat germ and another of granulated lecithin after every meal (these will keep the cholesterol level in its place, the triglycerides, as well as the blood pressure, along with other benefits).

14. Exercise from 20 to 30 minutes a day. It is not recommended to stress your body with hours of exercise, but you do have to be constant to see results and maintain at an optimal health condition. It would be ideal that with time you can reach the point when you can exercise from 45 to 60 minutes a day, 4 to 6 times per week. This is possible with discipline and consistency.

IMPORTANT: If you have never eaten healthy, it is probable that you are lacking discipline when eating, and discipline is difficult to achieve overnight, but there is an effective way of achieving it: Focus on the number 1 habit of this list, and until you have formed this habit, go to number 2, then number 3, then 4, etc... When you least expect it you will have acquired strong discipline and good habits.

TIPS ON HOW NOT TO GET STUCK WHILE LOSING WEIGHT

1. Self-sabotage is prohibited! Don't trick yourself by saying, "No one saw." Or, "I only ate two cookies." Or, "I am going to replace my salad with ice cream."

2. Don't buy foods that tempt you; keep junk food out of your house.

3. When you eat out, choose what you will eat wisely and never eat everything they serve. Don't eat bread with butter or chips with salsa, ask the waiter to take them away. While you wait for your food at a restaurant, talk with your dinner partner about your improvements since you started losing weight and thank him/her or thank each other because good nutrition benefits everyone. If your partner does not support you, look for another. In other words, look for a friend who has the same interest in nutrition as you do so that you can support each other. Motivation is vital in order to reach any goal.

4. Don't drink alcohol, not even 1 drink—that is—if you want to lose all your extra pounds. Once you have reached your goal you can drink from time to time (as an example, every 2 weeks).

5. Eat less than what you eat now and you will realize that 15 minutes after you eat, you will feel satisfied and full with

out the sensation that you have over-done it. It takes the brain 20 minutes to recognize you are full.

6. Don't forget that in order to keep losing weight you must get rid of all the toxins in your body. How? By drinking water and exercising.

7. Exercise! If you don't like it, at the very least find a sport that you enjoy and makes you sweat. Without exercise it will be harder to lose the last few pounds and if you don't work out on a regular basis, your muscles will be flaccid.

8. Stress makes you gain weight especially around the stomach. Not only that, but it wears out tissue (muscle); acidifies your blood; ages you; and slows down your metabolism. Control your stress by praying, working out, meditating, doing yoga, Pilates, dancing, walking or participating in sports etc...

9. Stop taking prescription anti-depressants because they affect your hormonal and metabolic systems. Instead, take vitamins, work out, drink water and eat healthy. Consider donating one or two hours of your time to nursing homes, orphanages or hospitals so that you can prove (to yourself if to no one else) that helping others without expecting anything in return helps cure depression. It is possible that doing this will help you stop thinking in your own problems, especially if they didn't have solution or if they are never going to happen. Make a list of the things that you don't like with regards to your personality and another list with all of the problems you currently have due to a lack of discipline. Organize this in an order of importance and each day at least try to resolve 1 of these problems. When you least expect it you will advance incredibly; otherwise the list of problems will grow. Nothing will magically disappear. If you can't do this on your own, get help.

10. Never compare yourself to your neighbor or your best friend. Everyone's skeletal system is different. Nature made some of us taller or thinner than others; or flatter or bulkier than others.

But what we do have in common is that if we don't watch what we eat, we all are going to get sick. So, your only competition should be with yourself.

11. Don't weigh yourself too often. As long as you know you are eating what you are supposed to, when you are supposed to, you are guaranteed to lose weight. Remember, you should be eating healthy foods including a variety of fruits, vegetables and whole grains. You also should be eating small animal protein portions and as long as you are digesting them properly without constipation or digestive problems, you will continue losing weight. Do not become obsessed by trying to lose weight all at once in the beginning; that makes you brain's chemistry change and blocks your metabolic system. Remember that it did not take your body a couple of months to gain dozens of pounds. It took it a lot longer, so it stands to reason that permanent weight-loss in a healthy manner also will take time, patience and discipline.

12. Raw vegetables can help you curb your appetite. And because they are water vegetables (over 80% water), they help detox the body and burn fat faster.

13. Varied green, raw vegetable juices nurture your organism directly and soothe your anxiety attacks for refined sugars and flours. They help you digest your food better. A better digestion helps you get rid of intestinal waste and avoid inflammation. The better you digest foods the faster you will lose weight.

14. Any health problem you may have interferes with your weight loss even if you are eating healthy because the food nutrients are first used to make the body well and then to burn fat.

15. Do you have health problems? Then a way to help your body heal itself—besides feeding it at the right times—is giving it all the nutrients it needs. If heat destroys some of those nutrients, pesticides destroy some more, and then your stress destroys some more... Can you imagine the vitamins that are left in these foods? These vitamins are a minimal amount of what

the body needs to function and heal itself. This is where B complex supplements, minerals, essential fatty acids, amino acids and enzymes come in.

16. Be grateful with life. Stop looking at the negative. Focus on what you do have and stop focusing on what you are missing. Be more thankful with what you have. Take advantage of what you have and use it, instead of spending your time complaining about what you would like to have. Strive for what you want to have, if you know that it's attainable. If you know it's impossible and maybe even irrational to obtain, forget it and become more realistic.

17. For example, it would be irrational for a short person who is about 5'4" and is in his/her 30's to suffer because he/she is not as tall as Anthony Robbins who is 6'7". What is possible even at 5'4" is to be healthy, happy and content with your work, and to have a healthy family that loves and respects you. However, in order to have it you need to deserve it. Do you want a better job? Go to school, better yourself. Do you not want to sacrifice the time it would take to study and work every day, leaving only a few hours for yourself? Then don't complain. Be grateful with life, it will help you be happy and being happy stimulates the immune and metabolic systems. Being unhappy acidifies and activates your defense mechanism. When that happens, you can't lose weight.

IMPORTANT: Take digestive enzymes before each meal; 100mg coenzyme Q-10 per day, Omega3 after each meal, calcium with magnesium 1 capsule 3 times a day on an empty stomach, vitamins B, C, E, A, minerals and 50mg of zinc. Minerals and zinc are better absorbed if taken at night.

THE BENEFITS OF WHEY AND YOGURT

What is whey? Whey is a yogurt relative that has similar properties. It also acts as an organism purifier and is easy to obtain on a daily basis. In order to get whey all you have to do is squeeze the juice of a lemon on whole milk then when this separates and curdles you strain it. The liquid is the whey and the mass that comes out you can use as cottage cheese. Whey detoxifies and strengthens the immune system and it helps prevent cancer, as well as other illnesses that start in the intestines.

HOW TO PREPARE AND EAT WHEY

In a container put equal parts of yogurt and whey; add your choice of chopped fruit, two tablespoons of wheat germ and two tablespoons of mixed ground seeds. (Flax, sunflower, sesame and pumpkin seeds) Add a tablespoon of honey and mix it well. Drink it once per day but if you suffer from digestive problems then take it up to 3 times per day (honey only once per day).

HOW TO PREPARE FRESH HOME MADE CHEESE

Once the milk has separated after the lemon you have squeezed into it, let it sit for several hours until it curdles perfectly. Then strain it, separate the whey from the solid. Place the solid on a thin, clean cloth (cheese cloth) put all four corners together and let it keep distilling. Afterwards place the solid on a plate with some weight on top so that it is pressed into cheese form. This cheese is only good for two days because it has no preservatives, unlike those sold in supermarkets, so don't make big batches of it.

NATURAL YOGURT

Plain yogurt cures infections, diarrhea, constipation, ulcers and any illness associated with the intestines or the digestive apparatus. It is also recommend for people who suffer from migraines, acne, colitis, ulcers, skin problems, fatigue, nervousness and herpes. It is also recommended that those who are lactose-intolerant replace cow milk with plain yogurt, since the microorganisms in yogurt destroy milk's protein molecules. These protein molecules cause the allergic reactions when you drink the milk. The somewhat acidic flavor of plain yogurt does not mean that your own stomach acids are going to get worse. On the contrary, yogurt will stop the production of excess of hydrochloric acid (digestive acid), which causes discomfort.

In order for plain yogurt to help lower cholesterol in the blood, you must use skimmed milk in its preparation. Plain yogurt is healthier than milk because of its nutritional and healing properties and low sugar levels.

It is known that the use of most antibiotics destroys intestinal flora and in order to replace it, you must consume natural foods such as plain yogurt, fruits and vegetables. If someone in your family suffers from a tumor, take the right measures to avoid getting this hereditary illness. The first thing you have to do is to eliminate red meats from your diet and increase your use of fruits, vegetables, seeds, nuts and sprouted grains.

HOW TO PREPARE YOGURT

First of all you must be super-clean when preparing yogurt to avoid contaminating it. If you have high cholesterol or are obese, use skimmed milk to make your yogurt and drink it every day. If you have anemia, malnutrition and even the tuberculosis virus, add one cup of cream for every liter of whole milk.

Warm up the milk until it starts to boil, then transfer it to a clay or glass container and let it cool off. Once it is lukewarm add the cream until it dissolves; if you don't need the cream, skip to the next step. Then, add a glass of plain yogurt or yogurt seed (this seed can be found in health food stores) and move it around slowly. Cover the container, wrap it in a warm towel and let it sit for 6 hours. If you would like for the yogurt to clot further, you can let it sit for another 6 hours.

NOTE: Keep a glass of yogurt aside so that you can use it in the next yogurt preparation the following day. If at any time the yogurt becomes insipid, begin the process once again.

CALCIUM

98% of the almost 3 pounds of calcium in the human body can be found in the bones, 1% in the teeth and the other 1% in tissues and the blood stream. Calcium and magnesium are the minerals that the body needs most. It uses up calcium twice as much as other minerals. With the help of magnesium, calcium takes care of the proper operation of the blood, nerves, muscles and tissues; it especially regulates heart and muscle contractions.

When the calcium level in our tissues is low, the body takes calcium out of our bones. But when we have an excess of calcium due to synthetic calcium or lack of magnesium, the body sends it to the wrong places like artery plaques or to joints, muscles or the liver and the blood, causing inflammation and disabling pain.

Why does alkaline blood become acidic? It happens when we eat whatever, however without caring if it is junk or not. Alkaline blood will also become acidic due to continuous constipation, excessive consumption of refined carbs (white flours and refined sugars) and an excess consumption of red meats.

This problem of acidosis in the blood is considered an illness of the immune system. Eating healthy improves digestion and prevents intestinal flora leaks. Flora is essential in preventing allergies and arthritis pain.

THE BENEFITS OF CALCIUM

Calcium reduces headaches, irritability, insomnia, and depression. In women, calcium reduces premenstrual, pre-menopause, menopause and post-menopause symptoms. In men, it reduces andropause (male menopause) symptoms. It is beneficial to take high calcium dosages for short periods of time. The best way to take calcium is on an empty stomach at night and with a betaine capsule. It is recommended that those taking 2000mg of calcium with magnesium take 2 capsules on an empty stomach in the morning and 2 at night 1 or 2 hours before going to sleep.

WHO NEEDS TO TAKE MORE CALCIUM?

From pregnant women to lactating women; smokers, alcoholics, those who work out; sick, nervous or apprehensive people; those who consume high levels of protein, sugar, salt, or saturated fats and those who suffer from gastrointestinal problems need more calcium than others.

The kidneys must be in good working condition in order to control the calcium level in the blood. If they do not work properly, the calcium will go to the blood instead of to the bones. In order to take good care of your kidneys, all you have to do is drink 2 or 3 liters of water. Remember that the kidney's job is to purify the blood and filter out toxic substances from the body.

Calcium is vital for adolescents; females starting at 12 years of age and males starting at age fourteen. During a 3 or 4 year period, adolescent bodies need more calcium because it is during that period of life that 40% of the bone forms that they will have for the rest of their lives. Calcium is absorbed in the small intestine with the help of magnesium and vitamin D.

Children and adolescents need 200 IU of vitamin D per day. But 90% of all adolescents, especially young women, do not consume calcium, not even the minimum doses. They prefer sodas and juices instead of milk and vegetables. Many youngsters believe that milk is fattening when in reality what makes you fat are all the chemicals in diet sodas and the concentrated sugar in commercialized juices. These drinks are not only fattening and intoxicating, but they rob the calcium and minerals from the bones.

THINGS THAT REDUCE CALCIUM ABSORPTION

- High salt diets cause calcium loss.

- High sugar diets reduce calcium and magnesium absorption.

- Synthetic calcium or without magnesium adds up to a calcification of soft tissue, formation of kidney stones, calcification of the skeletal bones and hypercalcemia (high levels of calcium in the blood).

- Toxins found in cigarettes, alcohol and in recreational and prescription drugs hinder calcium absorption and as a consequence, rob the bones of their calcium reserves.

- High animal protein diets, like the Atkins Diet acidify the organism's tissue and blood; in the attempt of preventing the perforation of organs due to excess of acids, the body lets go of the calcium in the bones in great quantities. The result of this process is an increased risk of osteoporosis, arthritis and other autoimmune diseases. This type of diet also causes the loss of sodium in the body; remember that calcium and sodium both use the same means of transportation and where calcium goes so does sodium.

• Stress affects body homeostasis (balance). This balance is kept through calcium levels and the operation of the thyroid gland, which in turn is in charge of the production of vitamin D and the hormones parathyroid, calcitonin and dihydroxide.

• Calcium absorption prevents gastrointestinal problems since calcium is absorbed in the small intestine with the help of magnesium and vitamin D.

• Diets high in phosphorous and low in calcium result in bone calcification. They also lower calcium and mineral absorption. Phosphorous is found in soda, meat, eggs, and processed foods, deli meats like sausage, ham, bacon, etc... and in all creamy cheeses.

• People who suffered fractures in their childhood have increased difficulty absorbing calcium; and if during their adolescence they had poor eating habits and did not take care of their bodies, they also run the risk of having problems with their bone system throughout their adult life.

• Skimmed milk interferes with calcium absorption. Foods high in oxalic acids such as spinach, rhubarb, chard and chocolate (this acid forms insoluble salts in the intestine) have the same effect.

• Milk fortified with vitamin D is not recommended because since it is synthetic vitamin D, it also interferes with calcium absorption.

• Phytic acid also diminishes calcium and mineral absorption. Whole grains have this acid as well; this is why it is recommended they be soaked for 24 to 48 hours before cooking.

IMPORTANT: Porous, fragile bones and calcium loss occur when calcium is used up faster than the body can replace it. And all the points already mentioned above interfere with the calcium absorption to wear it down faster than the body is able to deposit new calcium.

PHYSIOLOGICAL REQUIREMENTS

Everyone needs calcium! Little ones, big ones, men and women included. But the amount each person needs depends on the physiological requirements of the body during its development. This has to do with age, gender, physical activity, lifestyle and nutrition.

CALCIUM DOSES ACCORDING TO AGE

The best source of calcium for newborns up to age 1 is breast milk. During the first 6 months, a baby who drinks breast milk gets about 360mg of calcium per day. After the first 6 months, once a baby begins eating solids, a baby must consume about 540mg of calcium per day. It is not recommended that babies consume solids before 6 months of age because their digestive and immune systems are still not fully-developed. Feeding solids to a baby before 6 months of age can lead to food and environmental allergies well into adult life.

Calcium found in breast milk is 58% more easily absorbed than calcium found in baby formulas. Cow's milk is not recommended until the child turns 12 months old. However, plain yogurt, whey and tofu can be included in a baby's diet from 6 months of age.

From age 1 to 3 years, children need around 500mg of calcium.

From age 4 to 8 years, they need around 800mg. From 9 to 18 years of age they need 1300mg of calcium per day. If you ingest too much calcium the body will simply eliminate the excess. But if growing children do not get enough calcium, the bones in infants and adolescents don't grow as they should. Not only that, but the bone becomes weak, vulnerable and fragile.

Adults 19 to 50 years of age need at least 1000mg of calcium per day. Pregnant or lactating women need at least 1200mg per day. Pre-, post- and menopausal women need 1200mg of calcium with magnesium; this if you are not taking estrogen. Since the body of a young person absorbs 50 to 70% of the consumed calcium, while adults and elderly people only absorb 20 to 50% of the ingested calcium, it is recommended that you are conscious of what you eat and that you take extra calcium in a supplement form.

For people who have health problems or smoke, drink alcohol, coffee or soda and whose lifestyle is sedentary or stressful, it is recommended they take 2,000 to 4,000mg of calcium per day. If you will be taking large doses of calcium make sure you let your body rest every three months for 1 or 2 weeks and then continue your treatment. In order for the body to truly absorb the calcium, it must come in a formula that contains magnesium, vitamin D, zinc and other minerals in smaller doses. Calcium taken alone can be counterproductive.

INTOLERANCE TO COW'S MILK

Intolerance of sugars found in cow's milk—lactose—occurs due to a lack of the enzyme that digests it. People of African, Mexican, Indian-American and Asian descent, genetically tend to suffer more of lactose intolerance. Anyone who cannot digest lactose can

improve this condition through nutrition by fortifying the immune system and repairing the intestinal flora.

Stop attacking your immune system with chemicals and artificial colors found in prepackaged food, fast food, canned food, fried food and artificial food. Reduce the toxins in cigarettes, alcohol, coffee, prescribed or street drugs and sugars. Lastly, in order to repair your intestinal flora and fortify your immune system, let you digestive apparatus rest and take calcium. Eat 3 or 4 small portions of foods that contain calcium every 3 hours.

NOT ONLY COW'S MILK HAS CALCIUM

If you are the kind of person who has decided not to drink cow's milk, don't worry. Calcium can also be found in many other foods and a rotating diet can get them going for you. Here are some alternatives and their content of calcium:

- 6 oz. of plain yogurt contains
300mg of calcium

- 1 cup of steamed broccoli contains
250mg of calcium

- 6 oz. of goat milk contains
240mg of calcium

- 6 oz. of steamed collard greens contains
255mg of calcium

- 6 oz. of turnips with roots and leaves cont.
220mg of calcium

- 3 oz. of almonds contains
210mg of calcium

- 3 oz. of tofu contains
110 mg of calcium

- 1 ½ oz. of parsley contains
80 mg of calcium

- ¼ cup of kelp contains
80 mg of calcium

- 2 oz. of sunflower seeds contains
80 mg of calcium

- 2 oz. of sesame seeds contains
75 mg of calcium

NUTRITION AND CALCIUM

Replace cow milk (it irritates the membranes and joints more) with soy milk or plain yogurt. Increase your use of raw vegetables and ripe fruits especially cantaloupe.

Avoid eating wheat, cow's milk, tomatoes, potatoes, eggplant and bell peppers, as these foods irritate membranes and joints.

The acidity in the blood also causes water retention because the body needs extra water to dilute the acid excess in the blood and that is how it keeps these acids from destroying internal organs.

Deep breathing equalizes the body's chemistry while it gives red blood cells more oxygen and eliminates carbon dioxide through exhalation. Rest, positive thoughts, fresh air and exercise also help maintain the body's homeostasis or its chemical and blood acid balance.

Some alkaline foods necessary to neutralize acidic blood are raw vegetables and fresh ripe fruit. Acidic fruits such as pineapple and tomatoes eaten raw have alkaline effects after digestion. Carrot juice, watermelon and celery are also alkaline, as are unpasteurized honey, raw almonds, peanut butter and seaweed.

Soak dried fruits and seeds for 30 minutes before eating them. Soak oatmeal in water for 30 minutes and then discard the water so that you can re-boil it in new water. Soak legumes the night before cooking them or use the quick method: boil them for 1 minute, cover them and let them sit for 1 hour then toss the water and cook them in new water.

NOTE: Canned foods and foods with additives acidify the blood. Most cereals are acidic except those made with sprouted grains. Eating fruits and vegetables help calcium absorption thanks to the potassium and bicarbonate that we find in them. Potassium and bicarbonate can diminish the hypercalciuric effects (rapid calcification of the blood) in diets high in sodium and chloride.

People who have worked out since they were little suffer less bone system and calcium retention problems. It is better to run and jump when you are young than it is to swim. Swimming is great but in order for the bones to grow strong you must use them.

People who have suffered obesity since they were children run a higher risk of sustaining fractures or bone diseases in their adult life. That's why you should help and motivate your child to work out even if he/she is not obese. It also stands to reason that if he/she does have some extra pounds, establishing a regular routine of working out is even more important. Set the example by working out and ask him/her to join you, so you can improve your weight and health together.

SMOOTHIES HIGH IN CALCIUM (500mg) AND ESSENTIAL MINERALS

- ¼ Cup of whey

- 1 Cup of plain liquid yogurt (kefir)

- 4 oz. of frozen or fresh multi-berries and 1 Date

- 1 pkg. of stevia sweetener and 1tsp. of pistachios or 6 almonds

- 1 Tbsp. of mixed ground seeds

- 2 Tbsp. of natural raw oatmeal

Put it all together in a blender, mix and it's ready.

NOTE: Whey can be obtained squeezing 2 big lemons in 1 liter of cow milk. Let it sit for 1 1/2 days and once the milk curdles, the transparent liquid is the whey and the solid is cottage cheese.

Mixed ground seeds can be made by placing dry sunflower, sesame, pumpkin and flax seeds in the blender. After grinding each kind of seed separately in the blender and in equal amounts, you can mix them together and store them in a glass or plastic container with a lid.

WARNING: Chocolate milk (for the chocolate shake lovers), does not allow the body to absorb calcium. So don't forget to eat foods high in calcium and/or take a calcium supplement.

CARBOHYDRATES

Carbohydrates are the most important nourishment for our bodies because they are the main source of energy for life. In a healthy diet, 60% of calories have to come from carbs. Most people focus more on protein than carbs. Almost everyone believes that carbs make you fat, but that is not so. On the contrary, protein cannot build more muscle mass without carbohydrates.

First you must know what carbs are. The easiest way to see it is by describing several sugar molecule chains of different sizes, some are long; others are short. Short sugar molecule chains are basically simple carbs and the long chains are complex carbs. Carbohydrates are sugars and starches that the body converts into glucose or fructose. It doesn't matter what kind of carbs you eat they all become glucose so that the body can use it as energy.

A small glucose portion becomes glycogen in order to be stored in the liver and the muscles. The rest of the glucose generated by the body becomes fat stored in fat cells.

4 TYPES OF CARBOHYDRATES

There are 4 types of digestible carbs which are very important to identify for the health of your body.

- NON-REFINED COMPLEX CARBOHYDRATES

These generally are high in vitamins, minerals and fiber, but low on the glycemic index (low in simple sugars). You can find them in brown rice, whole grain breads and cereals, sweet potatoes, red potatoes, beans, oatmeal and vegetables.

- REFINED COMPLEX CARBOHYDRATES

These are generally processed carbs high in the glycemic index (high simple sugars). They hardly have any fiber, vitamins or minerals and they are digested rapidly; this is why you get hungry in short time after consuming foods with refined complex carbs. These carbs are found in white rice, white bread, tortillas made with refined flour, bagels, russet potatoes and refined cereals.

- NATURAL SIMPLE CARBOHYDRATES

Carbs high in the glycemic index (too much simple sugar) include natural simple carbs found in fresh fruits and fruit juices. The sugar from these kinds of carbs are absorbed easily, which is why you should consume small portions of fresh fruit and that you drink only 4 ounces of juice right after making it.

- PROCESSED SIMPLE CARBOHYDRATES

High on the glycemic index (too much simple sugar), processed simple carbs can be found in sweet drinks, commercial fruit juices, sodas, pastries, donuts, marshmallows, lollipops, ice cream and other sweets. These carbs are immediately absorbed by the body and its negative effects can be felt in a matter of minutes (hyperactivity, sugar crash, anxiety, hunger and sugar cravings, irritability, fatigue and nervousness).

CAUTION: When you consume carbs—good or bad—they give you immediate energy. But the bad carbs take twice as much from you, and the energy they return only lasts 30 minutes. If you eat good carbs, these also give you immediate energy, but this energy lasts hours and the best part is that with them you won't experience sugar crashes, fatigue, anxiety, sugar cravings and irritability.

Now that you know about these different types of carbs, let's take a look at the positive and negative relationships between diabetes and carbs. Good and bad carbs become glucose in the body; glucose is the sugar in the blood. Without sugar in the blood, the brain cannot function so it is necessary to have glucose in the blood stream.

Each gram of carbs has 4 calories, and if we don't use them during the day because "**we did not have time to exercise**", our bodies can only burn 60% of the calories consumed from carbs (used to keep us alive). This percentage is based on the 1,800 calories we are supposed to consume daily. If you eat 3,000 calories from carbs, 1,000 calories from protein and 1,000 calories from fat, your total in a day easily can reach 5,000; far more than recommended. This produces a great strain on your liver and pancreas. Do you know how many calories you are eating per day?

A medium-sized chocolate bar has between 200 and 300 calories. The Nutritional Content Chart says that the average chocolate bar is enough for three people. Just how much of that bar do we actually eat by ourselves? All of it, right? So, we end up eating about 1,000 calories and if to this we add a pastry with a cup of coffee in the morning, (about another 120 calories) then a piece of fruit (50 calories) later a hamburger (700 calories), fries (200 more calories), when choosing something to drink, we tell ourselves that at least the soda is "diet" right? But we ignore the fact that even if diet soda does not have calories it does have cancer-causing chemicals. We have not reached dinner yet and we have already consumed about 2,000 calories.

If we decide to have *carne con chile (meat with chili sauce)*, rice, refried beans and tortillas for dinner, we will be adding at least some 900 to 1,200 calories (depending on the portion sizes) to what we've already consumed during the day, then if someone brings out the ice cream . . .

Oh no! Let us add the 2,070 calories from the foods we ate during the day to the 1,500 calories from dinner, and it all comes to 3,570 calories. Remember that we only burn 60% of 2,000 calories derived from carbs. These are the only ones our bodies will process. The rest we'd have to burn off at the gym, running around our house, or skipping rope in the living room. If we don't exercise, then all these extra calories become fat, cellulite and toxins. Not only will we gain weight and clothing sizes, but the levels of fat running through our bloodstream (cholesterol and triglycerides) will also increase. This type of fat causes cardiovascular problems, diabetes, depression, chronic fatigue, sexual impotence, and skin problems just to name a few of its most destructive effects.

Whether you get diabetes due to high levels of glucose or sugar, or low levels of these give you hypoglycemia, these problems will become chronic and may cause death. Adrenal and pancreatic hormones: adrenaline and insulin are extremely important to metabolize sugar. When you eat excessive quantities of refined carbs, glucose levels in the blood and tissue lose their balance.

Even sugar that comes from fruit must be monitored in order to avoid large quantities of glucose in the blood, all types of sugar whether refined or sugar in fresh fruit goes directly to the blood increasing the risk of diabetes.

Did you know there are people addicted to bad carbs? Of course! Generally people who suffer from this addiction are also over-weight and suffer from high blood pressure, high cholesterol, and even diabetes. This is why a lot of people believe carbs make you fat, but they actually don't, people that abuse them are the ones that gain weight. Most women think that bread and tortillas make them fat. So, instead of moderating their consumption of these foods, they stop eating them entirely.

An extreme: the addiction to refined carbs. Another extreme: starving oneself by avoiding all carbs in order to lose weight. Not eating carbs can help you lose weight quickly, but lets not get confused! The bad carbs we must avoid are refined carbs; we gain weight when we eat these in large portions. The next time you tell yourself, "I'm going to stop eating carbs", just say, "I'm going to stop eating refined carbs". The carbs in breads made out of whole grain or sprouted grains and vegetables are vital in order to avoid colon cancer, malnutrition, and anxiety attacks. The less anxiety attacks you have, the easier it will be to gain nutritional discipline.

This is why extreme diets don't work. The "protein" diet as an example, how long do you think you would be able to avoid eating bread, tortillas, cereal, vegetables, and fruit? Our common sense should tell us that this diet is not healthy and that something bad will happen to us if we follow it for too long.

WHAT TYPES OF CARBOHYDRATES SHOULD WE EAT?

The beast carbs are: complex carbs found in fruits, brown rice, vegetables, oats, beans, bread, and whole grain and germinated-grain tortillas, etc... Brown rice has fiber, minerals, no fat and not too much sugar. This is why brown rice is much healthier than white rice for your health in general. If you need carbs right after your workout, there's nothing better than fresh fruit.

THE DISADVANTAGE OF REFINED CARBOHYDRATES

The main problem with snacks made from refined carbs is that they are high in starches and simple sugars, low on vitamins, minerals, and fiber; worst of all, they can suddenly spike your sugar level. When the sugar level is too high, insulin immediately goes to the rescue, and when insulin consumes so much sugar at a time you feel the effect: fatigue, dizziness, nervousness, headaches, sugar cravings, and worse of all, it eliminates your appetite for healthy foods.

WHAT IS IN THE SODA AND COMMERCIAL FRUIT JUICES?

You have to get used to reading the labels of what you eat and drink. If you pay attention, a soda or a commercial fruit juice has around 50 grams of carbs, and guess what refined carbs means on the label? Correct... additives, sugars, and calories. So basically you are drinking water with 50 grams of sugar and a stack of chemicals and artificial flavors. Did you know that cola sodas are used by CHP officers to remove blood stains from the concrete after car accidents? Did you know that for over 20 years, citric and phosphorous acids have been used to clean heavy machinery and car batteries? All sodas, light and dark contain these types of acids. Put this to the test; place a nail in dark soda for 4 days and see what happens to that nail. It disintegrates!

Next time you wish to clean your bathroom and remove sediment from your bathtub, just apply some dark soda and let it sit for a few hours. Imagine what these chemicals are doing to your internal organs, worse yet, to your children's bodies.

HOW HEALTHY IS COMMERCIAL YOGURT?

We watch commercials on TV that use thin models eating yogurt supposedly to lose weight. If you read the labels on commercial flavored yogurt you will see that each portion has about 40 grams of carbs and 25 grams of sugar; these carbohydrates will convert to sugar. What you are basically eating are 65 grams of curdled sugar. This type of sugar (lactose) causes fatigue, intestinal inflammation, gas, and abdominal pain in most people.

CARBOHYDRATES AT NIGHT

All types of carbs—even healthy ones— are converted into sugar that then is stored as fat. Another reason to avoid carbs at night is that if you don't, you'll go to bed with high levels of insulin and it is guaranteed that your body won't be able to burn fat while you sleep. Also, when insulin levels go down, generally it wakes you up, making it difficult to get back to sleep.

If you're trying to burn fat and keep your muscle tissue, then you must take advantage of the GH (grown hormone). This hormone is released in the body during the first 90 minutes of deep sleep while blood sugar levels are low. The GH hormone also handles gradual fuel exchanges the body uses and during these first 90 minutes of deep sleep, the body uses more fatty acids than glycogen and protein. So, if you eat carbs before bed the GH hormone won't be released. This is precisely why body builders do not take any carbs at night. Nutrition recommends you have diner 3 hours before bed time.

IMPORTANT: The GH growth hormone is also activated after the first 15 or 20 minutes of working out. Once it is activated it starts using fat as a source of energy; so if you want to lose weight, keep working out for an additional 20 to 25 minutes. Make sure you also drink water while you are training.

FRIED FOOD

WHY AVOID FRIED FOOD?

Did you know that the fat from fried foods delays digestion for up to 20 hours? Imagine your stomach with food stuck in there for so many hours! You have not yet digested the chicken and fries from a couple of hours ago before you eat again. What do you think happens to the undigested food? Very simply, it is decomposing and putrefying, accumulating gases and toxins in the colon and large intestine.

With fatty acids and natural fats the process is entirely different. When we ingest fats in their natural state, such as dressings made with olive, sesame, or grape seed oil or we eat nuts, almonds and avocados, this type of fat has the same chemistry as our bodies. This is why the body quickly recognizes and processes it to use as energy when it needs it. Fat helps our digestive apparatus process the nutrients from foods and at the same time gives us energy; but only natural fats not saturated or hydrogenated fats in fried foods. Next time you see an exquisitely-fried dish, just picture it stuck in your stomach for 20 hours and rotting away in there. Grape seed and avocado oils are the best to cook with because they don't burn and can hold up to 490 degrees of heat without losing their properties.

WHAT IS HIDDEN SATURATED FAT?

Hidden saturated fat is also known as trans-fat. These trans-fats or in this case hidden saturated fats are used in the hydrogenation of oils used to fry food or used in the baking of cookies and pastries.

HYDROGENATION OF OILS

When fats or oils are hydrogenated, the molecular structures of the fats change. This change makes the oil become solid, hard and creamy, which makes it easier to store and keep longer.

HYDROGENATION PROCESS

Oil is heated and put under pressure for hours with hydrogen gas and with the help of a metal called nickel. The hydrogen and carbon atoms are what help the oil become creamy and solid. Then to finalize the process, this solidified hydrogenated fat is then filtered and whitened with chemicals. This is almost the same as how plastics are made! The end result is completely different from the oil that was used in the beginning of the process—so different in fact, that the process ends up destroying essential fats such as Omega 3 and 6 (the healthy component of oils).

NOTE: as of January 1 2006, it has been mandatory in the United States that food labels identify foods containing trans-fats. So, look for words such as, "partially-hydrogenated", "vegetable oil" and "shortening" so that you may avoid these foods. The trans-fats in these hydrogenated and fried foods attach themselves to the arteries, blocking circulation and increasing the risk for heart attacks and all other types of cardiovascular diseases. These types of fats are also responsible for childhood obesity, chronic fatigue, sexual and hormonal dysfunctions, diabetes and other serious health problems in this country.

DETOXIFICATION

Questionnaire to measure toxin levels of the body:

1. Is your energy level low in the morning and then again at around 3:00pm?

2. Do you have bad breath or a bitter taste in your mouth most of the day?

3. Do you have a strong odor in your body and your feet?

4. Do you need to sleep more than eight hours each night?

5. Do you have a low tolerance of alcohol?

6. Are you more sensitive to the cold than others?

7. Do you often have a pain in the upper part of your right side near your ribs?

8. Do you have bowel movements less than once a day?

9. Is you fecal matter of a yellow color and have a bad smell?

10. Do you suffer of chronic constipation?

11. Do you have pain in your joints?

12. Is your skin dry, oily or does it have has dark spots?

13. Do you have more than two drinks containing alcohol per day?

14. Do you suffer indigestion when you eat fast food?

15. Do you get bloated when you eat onions, radishes, cucumbers, and cabbage?

16. Do you have poor appetite?

17. Are you frequently nauseated?

18. Do you have itchy skin?

19. Do you suffer from asthma, eczema, allergies and/or acne?

If you answered yes to between five and eight of these questions, it is likely that the toxin levels in your blood are high. If you answered yes to nine or more, you definitely have high levels of toxins in your body. You will now have to detox your blood, tissue and body organs. There are several ways you can rid your body of toxins.

In order to clean and detox your body, you must first stop eating foods with no nutritional value for a few weeks. If you choose to continue eating junk food, at the very least do so in moderation. Once your body begins ridding itself of the excess of toxins and neutralizing your digestive system then you can choose one of the following detox techniques:

• Once a week for the entire day have fruit, salads (with olive oil, sea salt and lemon), vegetables, almonds, seeds, green juices, and distilled water with lemon (no sugar). In other words, do the water diet one day a week; it is called the water diet because the fruit, vegetables, salads, and juices are considered water foods. If this technique is too difficult for you to follow, don't worry, here are other options.

• For 13 consecutive days or during 2 weeks, from the time you wake up until noon, eat only vegetables, drink vegetable juices with 1/2 a piece of fruit and drink water with lemon. What happens in this method is that starting at around 4:00 am until 12:00 noon; the body cleanses itself in a natural way. If you only have liquids with nutrients, the blood and the liver are detoxified a lot easier and at the same time you allow your digestive system to rest. Oh! But if you are planning on not eating or drinking anything until noon in an attempt to lose weight faster, you are wrong. Instead of burning fat and detoxifying yourself, you will waste and metabolize (destroy) muscle in order to provide energy for the body. So be careful with self-sabotage and don't cheat.

• You can also detoxify with an 8 ounce smoothie made with parsley, celery and cactus; drink this without straining for 18 days in the morning while fasting. Avoid citrus fruits (except lemon), chocolate, tomato (especially cooked), coffee, alcoholic beverages, fried foods, spices, peppers (*chili*), sodas, sugars and cigarettes.

OPTIONAL DETOXIFICATION METHODS

A detox meal plan can last from 3 to 13 days. People with eating disorders such as bulimia or anorexia, pregnant or lactating women or people currently taking prescription medication should check with their doctor or nutritionist before trying any plan. Once you start your detox program you will not be able to drink coffee, sodas, commercial water, anything with sugar, fat, alcohol or nicotine. You will even have to give up refined tea (except natural green, chamomile or red tea).

This diet is high in natural fibers, vitamin A and C, nutrients and antioxidants such as zinc and selenium (antioxidants are the number-one protectors against cancer). What you will eat from 3 to 13 days is dependent on how long it has been since your last detoxification.

Foods you can eat are brown rice boiled in water. Brown rice is very high in vitamin B and is one of the best complexes for removing toxins stuck to the intestinal walls. You will also have to eat all kinds of fruits, vegetables, and salads, legumes such as peas, green beans and even garbanzo beans, lentils and lima beans. Add nuts and raw almonds with no salt or additives, flax, chia and pumpkin seeds, also raw. If you can, buy organic fruits and vegetables. If not, make sure you wash them well; soak them in water for 15 minutes with a bit of apple cider vinegar and a bit of lemon juice, then rinse them before eating them. During the days of your detoxification you cannot eat red meat; only white fish, salmon and chicken breast should be on your plate, and no dairy product except plain yogurt, soy or almond milk.

DETOXIFYING FRUITS

APPLES: help stabilize sugar levels in the blood, lower blood pressure, and lower cholesterol and calm you appetite.

AVOCADOS: should be used 2 or 3 times per week and it has an excellent combination of essential fatty acids.

BANANAS: should be eaten once or twice a week as an excellent source of potassium and tryptophan, which helps you sleep.

GRAPES: are high in potassium and recommended for people with heart problems and poor circulation. They also help stop the formation of mucous in the intestinal flora and help cleanse skin, liver, intestines and kidneys.

KIWI: is a tasty fruit is an excellent source of antioxidants, vitamin C and helps mop out toxins from the free radicals.

MANGO: is high in papain enzymes, which help with the digestion of the excess of protein. It cleanses the blood stream and mitigates depression.

PEACHES: are high in 3 super antioxidants: beta-carotene, selenium and vitamin C. These antioxidants help destroy toxins and free radicals.

PEARS: are high in healthy carbs and fiber which makes them a natural source of energy. They prevent constipation and are high in folic acid and vitamin C.

STRAWBERRIES: are very high in vitamin C.

DETOXIFYING VEGETABLES

BEETS: A super-detox food, beets are high in minerals and sweep out the kidneys and liver trash like a broom. Because of its strong flavor, it is recommended that you drink it with carrot juice.

BROCCOLI: This vegetable is a very complete and nutritious vegetable high in chlorophyll (natural green color). It is one of the strongest defenses to protect the body from cancer especially in the esophagus, stomach, colon, lung, larynx, prostate, mouth and pharynx.

CABBAGE: Red and white cabbages have curative properties that help prevent colon cancer, prevent and heal ulcers, stimulate the immune system, kill bacteria and all types of viruses. They also clean the mucous membranes of the intestines.

CARROTS: Excellent for the digestive system and cleanse toxins from the eyes. Carrots are one of the principal vegetables with antioxidants that block cancerous cells in the lung, and pancreas. A raw carrot a day diminishes the chances of getting lung cancer by up to fifty percent even in ex-smokers; they lower cholesterol and prevent constipation.

CAULIFLOWER: A relative of cabbage and broccoli with similar nutritional value, cauliflower helps reduce the risk of cancer in the colon and stomach.

CELERY: The root of celery has alkaline properties that reduce blood acidity, detoxify the organism, and remove tissue toxins. It is high in potassium, maintains the proper balance of necessary fluids and minerals for the nervous and circulatory system.

ENDIBIE: Is high in folic acid and vitamin C.

CRESS: Is high in anti-oxidants, vitamin C, iron, and calcium. It stimulates the metabolic and digestive systems and helps eliminate mucus in the intestines.

GREEN LEAF LETTUCE: High in vitamins A, C, folic acid, minerals, calcium, and iron. It helps with intestinal and liver functions and helps you sleep better.

ONION, GARLIC, LEEKS: These vegetables are good for the circulatory system and heart. Eat them to increase good cholesterol, improve blood circulation, lower triglycerides (blood fat), and regulate glucose levels in the blood. They also serve as anti-bacterial agents, and improve bronchitis symptoms.

POTATOES: High in potassium and vitamin C. Use potatoes occasionally (2 or 3 times per week) because of their high sugar and starch content.

BELL PEPPER: High in fiber and vitamin C, excellent for constipation prevention, detoxification and rejuvenation.

BREAKFAST IDEAS

- Fruit salads: mix your fruits daily so you don't get bored of eating the same fruits every day

- Soy or almond milk with avocado and banana shake

- Muesli, bran or sprouted grain cereals with fresh or dried peaches

- Plain yogurt with fresh fruit and gluten-free toast

LUNCH IDEAS

- Brown rice with vegetable salad and 5 chopped almonds

- 1 baked potato with kidney beans and salad with lettuce, spinach, cucumber, tomato, and radish, lemon, a pinch of sea salt with a bit of olive oil

- Lentil and onion soup with vegetables and a salad

- Bean salad with different types of beans. Drain them and add celery, spinach or whatever vegetables you wish

- Garbanzo soup, a salad and vegetables

DINNER IDEAS

- Steamed salmon, broccoli and a salad with lettuce, cucumber, carrots, etc...

- Brown rice, salad and steamed or fresh vegetables

- Grilled chicken breast (no fat or skin) or soup with vegetables, a salad and vegetables

- Baked potato, grilled white fish, vegetables and a salad

- Brown rice or sprouted grain gluten-free pasta with vegetables such as carrots, celery, garlic, mushrooms and a salad

DESSERTS

After dinner, wait 30 minutes before eating desserts like these:

- Fresh fruit or tropical salad prepared with mango, papaya, kiwi, etc...

- Strawberries with soy cream

- Plain yogurt with fruit

- 1 quarter cup of pumpkin seeds, chamomile tea and 6 almonds or nuts

NOTE: Remember that the body detoxes naturally between 4:00am and noon. After 12:00 noon, you should continue to eat healthy so that the process of detoxification can continue more efficiently. The following 8 hours after 8:00pm are considered the "assimilation period". During this time, the body absorbs nutrients in the liver, burns fat and destroys toxins. Any meal consumed after 8:00pm will not be digested. Instead, it will obstruct the absorption of vitamins in minerals and your liver will not be able to burn fat. In order prevent you getting hungry after 8:00pm (especially if you go to bed very late), you must plan your meal times and make sure your dinner is 3 hours before bedtime. If you get hungry after 8:00pm resist and only drink water. Within 2 days, your digestive system will get used to it and you will not get hungry. If you work nights and sleep during the day, then the hour at which you wake up is when your day starts with breakfast.

EXERCISE VERSUS OBESITY

Whoever said that in order to be healthy and have a good figure you must be a gym rat? In order to have energy, burn fat and strengthen your muscles you need to increase your activity level so that when you lose weight your skin is firm, not loose. To achieve this all you need is 15 to 20 minutes of exercise. The secret to working out is to break a sweat 3 to 4 times a week. You need to exercise at least 60 minutes per week.

For example, if you break a sweat in a 15 minute exercise session, those 15 minutes are not enough to complete your 60 minutes per week. Instead, you would have to work out for 15 minutes 4 times per week. But if you need to work out for 20 minutes continuously to break out a sweat, then you must workout for 20 minutes 3 times a week. The idea is that once you are able to complete your minimal workout and see the positive physical and mental effects, you will be encouraged to increase the intensity and duration until you're able to work out for 45 to 50 minutes 4 to 6 times a week.

The most effective exercise for the body is that which is not strenuous, but continuous. For example, you can burn a higher volume of fat walking nonstop for 30 minutes than you can when you play tennis for 45 minutes, because when you play tennis you run a lot with a lot of energy, but you are also constantly stopping.

Another benefit of moderately working out is that it diminishes appetite while the brain releases more endorphins. Endorphins are naturally-occurring chemical hormones in the brain that help keep the nervous system calm and relaxed. When you exercise vigorously, the metabolism accelerates and hunger increases. This does not mean that you should keep your metabolism turned off. On the contrary, you need to accelerate it to the extreme. Your metabolism turns on and works well only if you eat at the right times, avoid chemicals, and work out.

The effects of working out consistently are cumulative. That is, even if the exercise you do is not much, the benefits accumulate if you keep at it consistently. When you work out for 20 minutes a day, your metabolism stays turned on, burning fat up for up to 15 hours afterwards, even while your body is resting. That is why consistent exercise is cumulative.

Be careful not to fall into the workout protocol because when this happens your body no longer burns fat. On the contrary, it will keep you in fear of not having enough energy to continue working out. That is to say, when you become obsessed with exercise and spend hours at the gym every day without proper nutrition for that kind of extreme exercise, your body's chemistry changes. Instead of burning fat for energy it will use bone and muscle.

When you begin to work out for the first time in your life you also begin to replace fat with lean muscle. This lean muscle grows if the exercise is consistent so that the body begins to burn fat faster with the help of this lean muscle. Even if you don't lose many pounds, given the fact that muscle weighs more than fat, you will still drop considerable clothing sizes.

Walking, cycling, yoga, Pilates, and swimming are only some of the types of good exercises that can help you tone your muscles.

1. Lie down on your back on a thin mat with yours hands facing down and raise your legs as high as you can without bending your knees, then bring them down slowly. Do 3 sets of 3 repetitions each. Gradually increase the repetitions of each set.

2. Stand with your back against a wall and squat down slowly as if you were to sit on a chair. Do 3 sets of 15 repetitions each. Gradually increase the duration of each repetition in each set.

3. Lie down on your back and place a tennis ball or an orange between your legs. Raise your folded legs up keeping the orange between the legs. Do 3 sets of 15 repetitions, gradually increasing the number of repetitions.

According to neuropsychology, psychophysiology and nutrition experts, exercise not only helps you lose weight and prevent illnesses, but it also rejuvenates your brain and improves attention, concentration and memory. So to prevent premature aging of the brain it is important to practice some sort of exercise on a regular basis. With age or premature aging the brain loses weight and some of its abilities.

At birth, the human brain weighs around 350grams. In the adult stage, it can weigh up to 1,500 grams, or about 1 1/2 kilos. However, after 30 years of age we start losing neurons—and the worse we eat, the less we exercise, the faster this happens. With continued loss, at age 70 your brain might weigh around 1 kilogram. People who work out moderately during their entire lives maintain a younger more complete brain.

Any impairment or sickness keeping you from your regular work out or walk doesn't mean there is nothing you can do about it. At the very least, it is recommended that you do breathing exercises to help oxygenate the cells in your body and brain.

Dedicate 3 to 5 minutes 2 or 3 times per day to practice this breathing exercise: inhale slowly, hold it for 7 seconds and then exhale slowly for another 7 seconds. Do this for 5 minutes.

Once it becomes a habit, gradually increase your sessions until you reach 15 minutes of breathing exercise daily. The energy you will gain from this is immediate and if you learn to breathe properly (deep breathing) throughout the entire day, you will benefit from this immediately and long term.

THE IMPORTANCE OF WARMING UP

It is extremely important to warm up your muscles before working out in order to truly reap the benefits. When you start working out the muscle tissue will immediately use the local fuel it is able to get, which is glycogen instead of fat.

You might start to work out without warming up, but in doing so, you would only be using the glycogen in the body; then just when you are about to start using your fat, your work out has already ended.

Even worse, if you accustom your body to use only the glycogen in the tissue, it will be harder to burn fat. How long does it take the body to use fat as fuel? Depending on your metabolism and genetics it can take from 10 to 20 minutes.

There is a growth hormone "GH" that is released by the pituitarygland; this hormone is in charge of allowing release of body fat as a source of energy.

To stimulate the production of this hormone you need to first warm up the body so that it will use up the glycogen in the tissue and liver.

This is why it is so important to warm up first.

You can start your work out by walking 10 minutes. Gradually increase your warm up period from 15 to 20 minutes, followed by your workout.

EXCLUSIVE FOR RUNNERS

To find a runner's club in your area, visit www.rrca.org. Sometimes it's hard to get started, so motivation from other runners is extremely important to fulfill your wish of running a marathon someday.

Begin by walking and gradually increase your walking time. In order to avoid injury, you have to learn to listen to your organism; your body will tell you when you are ready to run your first mile. For 6 weeks, focus only on running that first mile you never thought you would be able to run.

After those 6 weeks, increase the intensity and training duration each week. If you can run 2 or more miles without fatigue several times a week, the heat of the moment will help you run the first 5 miles of your marathon—as long as you start off slow and maintain a steady pace.

WHY DO MUSCLES ACHE AFTER TRAINING?

The pain in your muscles after working out is the result of your muscle tissue tearing. Fortunately, the body's white cells and natural inflammation restore the damage done, which may last around 2 days in an otherwise healthy body.

You can use ice compressions to ease pain, eat healthy, drink plenty of water and get plenty of rest. Massages and liquids prepared with mint can help, but if you wish to be a marathon runner you must accept a certain level of pain as a natural part of the process.

After a recovery period, muscles become stronger. It is recommended that beginners don't do too much too soon. If your muscles continue hurting it might be because

a. You are not used to doing any kind of exercise

b. Your muscles are not used to this kind of training—maybe you changed your routine

c. You increased the intensity or duration of your training

DO YOU WANT TO RUN FAST?

If you want to run fast it is very simple; train and practice fast running. But be careful, because training too much all at once can be counterproductive. Signs that your body is running more than it should include loss of appetite, anxiety at night while trying to sleep and fatigue. These symptoms should disappear within 2 or 3 days without having to go to the doctor or without having to take any medicine for pain. You should lower the intensity or number of miles to your running routine.

If you are a beginner, it is recommended that you gradually increase the distance you run until you reach 4 to 6 miles per week. In order to increase resistance once a week, try to run as many miles as you possibly can. Running 3 or 4 miles is considered a long run for beginners. You have to stress the body just enough without overdoing it in order to achieve increased speed.

- Do not increase stress on your body too often. Wait 3 or 4 weeks so that your body can adjust.

- It is hard for your personal trainer or running partner to decide when you need to increase the intensity of your workout. But it is not hard for you to know if you will only listen to your body.

- Runners who train for long distance runs do not use all of the muscles necessary for sprinting.

- If you wish to become a sprinter, you still have to train and run long distances at normal speeds while continuing sprinting practice.

- The more oxygen enters your muscles the faster you can run.

- You get the most oxygen by training 70% to 80% of your MHR (maximum heart rate).

- If you train more than 85% of your maximum capacity, your body will use energy from the muscles. If you don't have enough oxygen in your organism your resistance will go down noticeably and so will your health.

- With moderate training your achievements and improvements will be gradual and noticeable. Best of all, you will gain strength and endurance without getting hurt.

- Remember that not all of us were born to be 5, 10, or 26km runners, so enjoy your own personal achievements.

- To increase resistance, train 35 to 45 minutes. More than 45 minutes of training slows progress, because it is hard to maintain the intensity and speed for such a long time.

Here is a sample training regimen for running:

Week #1

- Monday: walk or rest

- Tuesday: run 3 miles

- Wednesday: walk or rest

- Thursday: run 2 miles

- Friday: rest

- Saturday: run 3 miles

- Sunday: walk 60 minutes

Total: you ran 8 miles and you rested while walking (this gives you resistance)

Week #2

- Monday through Friday keep the same regimen as Week #1

- Saturday: increase your 1/2 a mile

Total: you ran 8 ½ miles

Week #3

- Monday through Friday keep the same regimen as Week #2

- Saturday: increase your run by ½ a mile

Total: you are now able to run 9 miles

These changes are minimal but consistent and gradual. This approach will help you increase resistance and in turn, resistance prepares you to run faster. Keep increasing your runs by ½ a mile every Saturday until you reach 6 miles. You will be able to do this because you are letting your body rest the rest of the week, not stressing it but pushing it until you are able to run 11 miles per week (not counting the time spent walking).

SHORT RUNS OR SPRINTS

Once you have the necessary resistance every time you run, your last mile during training can be used to gain speed. Run as fast as you can the first 20 seconds of every minute, then the other 40 seconds, run at a normal pace. Do this every minute for the entire mile. Once you are able to this without becoming overly agitated, increase the seconds of your sprints.

The goal is to be able to run at an 85 of your MHR (maximum heart rate) for 1 minute. But, if in the next minute you are not able to get your cardiac rhythm down to 100 or less, that means you are still not in shape for these types of races. In this case you should continue practicing without getting too tired for several months before trying it again.

GAIN VELOCITY WITH FLEXIBILITY

- During training: practice lifting your knees as high as possible while running.

- During practice: avoid running on your entire sole; instead, run with the tip of your foot. The weight should fall on half of your foot, under the bone that supports the toes. Toes must always point forward.

- Train uphill and downhill so that you gain strength, resistance and speed.

- Eat healthy so your muscles grow. More muscle means more speed, even if many don't believe it to be true. Of course this means, real—not synthetic muscle (read the section on muscles).

- Lift weights after running especially on the days you run moderately. It is true that in order to burn fat it is recommended that you run after lifting weights. However, in order for runners to gain speed and muscle, it is better to lift weights after running. Running is your priority.

- It is very important to get your rest: It is not recommended to run every day with the same intensity. Muscles gain strength when they rest, so recuperation is vital. On the days that you rest from running, you can walk or do moderate resistance exercise.

NOTE: Take essential fats such as Omega 3, Vitamin C, and calcium with magnesium and vitamins with minerals (follow the instructions on each bottle).

SPORTS NUTRITION

Sports nutrition is not that different from a plain and healthy balanced diet, but its needs are obviously greater. A person is considered a professional athlete when he/she works out at least 1 hour per day, or 2 hours 3 times per week. Training is important, but without a proper nutrition plan, it can't be effective. For every hour you work out you must eat 500 to 1,000 calories per day, depending on the kind of exercise, previous training and intensity of your workout program.

An athlete must eat 80 to 120 grams of protein depending on the kind of sport he/she practices. He/she must also focus on eating complex carbs like bread, tortillas, cereals and whole and sprouted grain pastas, fruits, vegetables and legumes. Athletes of all levels of ability must not abuse animal protein or fried foods in order to avoid acidifying muscle tissue.

MISTAKES THAT MOST ATHLETES MAKE

It is a mistake to think that the base of an athlete's diet must be protein, because an excess of any 1 nutrient at the expense of others equally important is always counterproductive. For example; animal protein excess increases fat storage in the body, causes dehydration, kidney and liver problems and increase cholesterol, uric acid and ammonium.

REFINED CARBOHYDRATES

The amount of glucose that circulates in the blood is limited. That is why when you eat too many refined carbs (if there is nowhere to store them in glycogen form) the excess glucose (sugar) becomes fat. So, many athletes mistakenly think that they must not eat carbs, when in fact the carbs that must be avoided are the refined not the complex. If your diet is low in carbs you will suffer pre-exhaustion.

INCREASING THE STORAGE OF GLYCOGEN

Fat is important as a reserve, but it is better to increase the ability to store glycogen. The best way to increase glycogen storage is to stop working out and continue eating the same amount of carbs before returning to your workout routine. During the physical rest, the glycogen storage increases up to 70%. This technique is called carbo-loading. For example, if you train 2 to 3 times per week, it is normal for you to use up you glycogen reserves. In order to replace these reserves, you must eat enough complex carbs with some protein. Then, 3 days prior to the event, you must decrease training and increase complex carb consumption (bread, rice, beans, lentils, green beans, vegetables etc.). This lets glycogen deposits grow, and with it fatigue takes longer to show up. However, you must be careful not to become dehydrated in the process.

HOW TO PREVENT DEHYDRATION

When you begin to get thirsty during your training program it is a sign that you have already lost 1% of the sweat in your body. And if you don't hydrate soon, you will lose 2% of your water, at which point your performance will decline by 20%.

Becoming 8% dehydrated can cause a deadly heat stroke. In order to avoid this, you must drink 4 to 6 ounces of water every 15 to 20 minutes. The water must be lower than room temperature so that your rehydration is quick. When you sweat, you also lose electrolytes (minerals such as calcium, magnesium, potassium, sodium, etc...).

This is why it is important to replace them by drinking water with added electrolytes. For athletes (those who work out an hour a day) it is enough to drink 4 ounces of natural fruit juice (not commercial) or eat a fresh fruit after working out to replace the lost minerals. An athlete who works out 2 hours 3 times per week or one that runs more than 10 miles per week can replace lost potassium with just 6 ounces of natural fresh orange juice.

ARE SPORTS DRINKS HEALTHY?

Sports or isotonic drinks contain sugar in order to replace lost glycogen. Unfortunately, this energy is false, temporary and does more harm than good because eventually it causes fatigue and glucose crashes. It is better to drink natural fruit juices, water with electrolytes and eat fresh fruit.

ANTIOXIDANTS

Athletes expose their bodies to more free radicals than non-athletes. These free radicals shrink and age body cells, causing degenerative diseases. You must neutralize these free radicals with vitamin C, vitamin E, water with lemon, fruits, tomatoes and green, yellow and purple vegetables rich in antioxidants. Vitamin A is also an antioxidant found in carrots, fruits and red and orange vegetables.

Zinc and selenium are 2 minerals that help the body prevent cell oxidation during training. This valuable mineral is found in foods like meat, fish, eggs, vegetables and pumpkin seeds. Selenium can be found in cereals, onion, asparagus and plain yogurt.

CAFFEINE

Caffeine usage among athletes is very common despite controversy over its effects on the body. Caffeine stimulates adrenaline production (anti-stress hormone) and the adrenaline accelerates the release of fat from the body into the blood stream. This allows athletes to use muscle glycogen and fat as a source of energy, hence more resistance. Unfortunately, more than 2 cups of coffee per day also causes loss of resistance, headaches, dizziness, arrhythmia, insomnia and anxiety.

NOTE: A high dose of caffeine is considered a drug.

AMINO ACIDS

A healthy, balanced and organic diet with enough raw vegetables in it gives you all the vitamins, minerals and amino acids necessary to achieve optimum performance during athletic training. This is why it is usually not necessary to add amino acids. Eating something raw like 1/2 a cup of veggies and some fruit with any kind of protein helps the enzymes in the food become amino acids.

A multi-amino acid supplement after training for 6 weeks 3 or 4 times per year is more than enough to insure amino acid balance. Abusing this substance has more disadvantages than benefits.

These make you gain weight—but not because of an increase in muscle mass, like many might think. Instead, protein excess turns into fat and ammonium. Ammonium destroys tissue and bone and acidifies the body.

LACTIC ACID

It does not matter what kind of athlete you are or what your training routine is: when you work out too much your body will generate the famous lactic acid. All athletes, no matter how well they take care of themselves or how healthily they eat, make this acid—especially those who sprint. In order to neutralize this acid, sodium bicarbonate is recommended. After training, dissolve ¼ of a tablespoon sodium bicarbonate in a glass of water and drink it immediately.

NOTE: Take essential fats like Omega 3, vitamin C, vitamin A, vitamin E, calcium with magnesium, liquid chlorophyll, silica, glucosamine with chondroitin, MSM with vitamin C, vitamins with minerals, and zinc (look at your multivitamins, calcium or any other supplements that have minerals make sure you do not exceed 100mg of zinc per day).

FORMULAS TO FIND YOUR IDEAL WEIGHT

Men:

Ideal weight for men: 106 lbs. for the first 5' of height, plus 6 lbs. for each additional inch after that. For example, if you are 6'4" tall, your ideal weight should be according to this formula: 106 lbs. + 16" x 6 lbs. = an ideal weight of 202 lbs.

Another example: a man 5'11" should have an average weight of: 106 lbs. + 11" x 6 lbs. = 172 lbs.

Women:

Average weight for women should be calculated at 100lbs. for the first 5 feet of height and then 5 lbs. for each additional inch. For example, a woman 5'4" should calculate her average ideal weight in this way: 100 lbs. + 4" x 5 lbs. = 120 lbs.

A woman who is around 5'2" tall would find her average weight: 100 lbs. + 2" x 5 lbs. = 110 lbs.

IMPORTANT NOTE: This formula is only an average. You must remember that the bone structure of each person is different and makes your weight vary from 5 to 10 pounds, depending on your build.

In order to know if you bone structure is small, medium or large you can do the following:

Wrap your right hand around your left wrist. If you can touch the nail of your middle finger with the base of your thumb, your build is small. If you can only touch the tip of your middle finger with the thumb, then your build is medium. If there is a space between your middle finger and your thumb then your build is large. This technique can be used by men and women alike.

Keep in mind that age also has to do with your body structure; between 30 and 40 years of age, bone degeneration begins.

MISTAKES AND SELF-SABOTAGE

Mistake #1: Salads

For many, eating salads is the same as eating healthy but, how true is that idea? The answer is very simple: it depends on if you bought the salad; where you bought it; or, if you made the salad, how you prepared it.

98% percent of all salad bowls and burgers in a bowl purchased from fast food eateries are low in fiber and high in trans-fat, which is the worse one for your health since it clogs your arteries.

A crispy-chicken bacon ranch salad at one of these places has more calories and saturated fat than a hamburger: approximately 640 calories and 49 grams of fat. Compare that with the hamburger containing 600 calories and 33 grams of fat.

Keep in mind that 10% of the calories you eat must come from saturated fat (animal protein). That means that this kind of salad has all of the allowable saturated fats a body can metabolize in 1 day. This means that you will not be able to have milk, eggs, or any kind of meat for the rest of the day if you eat one of these salad bowls; instead, you could only eat vegetables, fruits and salads with no dressing and water.

Such salads are a poor choice, because they have hardly any fiber at all. Remember that fiber is like a broom and mop for the intestines to help prevent colon cancer and digestive problems including inflammation, abdominal pain, gases, constipation and diarrhea. Each person needs about 25 to 35 grams of fiber every day. Even so, many people eat refried rather than whole beans, thinking they're getting the necessary fiber in this way. The fiber crisis worsens when people refuse to eat the minimum recommended amount of veggies per day.

Some fast food restaurants serve a salad on a fried flour tortilla bowl. This salad has 13 grams of fiber—which is good—but it also has 42 grams of saturated fat and a lot of sodium (1,670mg). Compare that to the total amount of sodium our bodies can metabolize in a day, which is 2,400mg. In other words, after eating 1 of these salads, you would have to restrict yourself to eating foods with no salt the rest of the day to compensate. If you don't eat the tortilla or the dressing that comes with it, then the fat content would go down from 42 to 21 grams and the sodium from 1,670 to 1,400 mgs.

Mistake #2: The Weight Scale

Do you have "scale-phobia"? You are afraid of the scale but, you still weigh yourself twice a day? Well, it is recommended you weigh yourself once every 2 weeks while you are overweight and once per week after you have achieved your ideal weight.

Your weight varies day to day, and even hour to hour. If you weigh yourself with or without clothes, at morning, at night, before or after eating, before or after going to the bathroom, etc. your weight will always be different. That is why it is recommended you weigh yourself at the same time each day, with no clothes before breakfast.

A person who eats regularly healthy, moderate portions at regular times gains and loses 2 or 3 pounds daily. By contrast, a person who does not eat at regular times and does not watch what he/she eats could gain or lose 5 pounds from 1 day to the next. This effect has to do with water retention and water loss, is not the same as losing the fat.

Mistake #3: Weight-Lifting

Many women think that lifting weights is for men only because they do not wish to look masculine like those women that dedicate their lives to body-building.

Nonetheless, lifting weights is simply doing resistance exercise in order to strengthen the muscles and become stronger. A woman who lifts weights is not going to look like a man because the muscles in women are not as big as the muscles in men.

Women who have very muscular bodies may take male hormones and spend day and night at the gym. Let us remember that all stimulants like steroids and hormones put your life at risk.

Lifting weights helps women harden the muscle and discard toxins that contribute to cellulite. Since muscle is heavier than fat, weight lifting may not help you lose much weight, but since muscle takes up less space than fat, instead of losing weight you will noticeably reduce clothing sizes. Doing weights frequently and regularly helps you lose some weight faster.

A recent study showed that women who did resistance exercises or lifted weights for 25 weeks lost quantities of fat—especially around the stomach. Fat around the stomach is dangerous to keep because it increases the risk of cardiovascular diseases, heart attacks and diabetes.

You don't have to live at the gym or workout twice a day in order to see encouraging results. Lifting weights 2 or 3 times a week for 30 minutes and doing aerobic exercises 3 times a week for 30 to

45 minutes will not only help you lose weight, but also help prevent cardiovascular diseases and depression. The American Council for Exercise states that lifting "light weights" with multiple repetitions help tone and harden your muscles, while lifting "heavy weights" helps increase muscle strength and size.

Mistake #4: Ignoring Pain

Do you feel strong and tolerant to pain, or, are you simply too busy to listen to your body because work is more important to you? Physical pain is simply the way our body tells us that something is happening internally. Ironically, women go to the doctor more often but they take care of their bodies less well than men do.

When a man is sick, he's very whiny and immediately goes to bed to rest and will not do anything until he's better, but not a woman. The woman has too much work to do, and simply can't give herself that luxury.

A study of 1,725 women with ovarian cancer (one of the most dangerous because generally it is detected only once it has become very advanced) found that more than half of those women took more than three months to be diagnosed because even though they had many of the symptoms of a serious condition they did not make time to go to the doctor.

Those symptoms are: inflammation of the stomach, intestines and ovaries, pain in the abdomen and or pelvis, and bleeding.

Many other women with heart attacks have been experiencing symptoms of unusual fatigue and breathing problems for over a month and still do not go to the doctor.

Most of these women attribute their symptoms to menopause and age; others do not even mention these symptoms to their doctors.

Breast cancer is the second most common cause of death in young women and yet, breast cancer is one of the most easily-detected and preventable of all. Still, over 40% of women over the age of 40 in this country have not had a mammogram exam in the last year. Women over 40 should be checked annually, not only for breast cancer, but for other types of cancer as well.

So when your body uses pain to get your attention and lets you know something is not right, it is your responsibility to listen to it. Don't wait until it stops working to do something about it, because often by that time, it's too late.

Just think about the day that you get a heart attack. Even if you have all the obligations and work in the world you will be unable to do anything for yourself. Someone else will have to do all those things for you. And if you die, maybe your husband's new partner will have to handle your tasks because you will no longer be able to. So, it is better to miss a few days at work so you can take care of yourself and then return to your duties without worry. Would you rather miss a few days at work to return healthy, or continue working yourself so sick you can't return?

If you're the kind of person that says: "I don't like to miss work." Or, "I never take any days off so that my bosses are happy with me and won't fire me." Or, "I just don't have time". Big mistake! Your bosses may have to dismiss you if you get really sick—even if you're the nicest most punctual employee they may fire you without consideration. But when you do your job well and they value you, even if you take the days off you need to keep yourself healthy, and ask for a few more because you're sick and need them to recover fully, it is much less likely that you will get fired.

Mistake #5: Not Getting 8 Hours of Sleep

People who sleep only a little bit so that they can have enough time during the day to do all the things they want to get done end up paying a price for it; that price is good health. People who do that are only fooling themselves because if they don't eat and sleep well, even if they are awake and busy all day, they will not have the necessary energy to keep going.

On the other hand, when you sleep 8 hours you have the energy to do everything including eating at the right time. Many women say that staying up late is the only way they have time for themselves. But that time may not be well-spent because they don't work out, they don't read, or meditate. Instead they handle house chores like laundry and ironing.

Our bodies need at least 8 hours of rest in order to repair wear and tear caused by stress during the day. If you are sleepy during the day it is because you are not resting enough or eating well. If you're not sleeping eight hours per night for 10 years, your risk of having a heart attack increases. Those 8 hours of rest are also crucial in order to maintain a healthy weight. Failing to sleep at least 8 hours causes hormonal imbalances, weight gain, and slows down your metabolism.

According to studies, not sleeping 8 hours causes depression, anxiety, highs and lows in blood glucose levels, high blood pressure, heart problems and Type II Diabetes. Consider yourself at risk of causing an accident which cause serious injuries to 40,000 innocent people per year and death to another 1,500 people.

Solution:

Do not commit to do more than what you can in one day. Divide your responsibilities with the rest of your family or your partner. If you don't have one or the other, give yourself time to handle all the tasks you have and make a priority list. Test your discipline and establish a time to go to bed every evening at the same time. Then allow yourself time to wake up regularly each morning. Plan in advanced the things you're going to do, and if you don't have enough time, postpone them for the following day. Don't drink coffee and make sure you have something nutritious for breakfast to start your metabolism and burn accumulated fat. Do not drink alcohol at night even if you think it relaxes you. Better said—it does relax you but only for a while, then insomnia kicks in.

Mistake #6: Indulging in Extremes

Many people abuse junk food and when they find themselves in a corner at a dead end, they take extreme measures to see immediate results, going from one extreme to the other.

In nutrition it is much smarter to replace synthetic with natural, and refined with whole foods. Instead of not eating it is better to be aware of what you put in your mouth.

Here is a list of basic nutrition foods (grocery list) that I recommend so that you can gradually start replacing traditional bad eating habits with more nutritious alternatives.

- Instead of refined flours, have: bread, tortillas, cereals and pastas made of multi- or sprouted flourless grains.

- Instead of commercial oils and saturated fats for cooking, use grape seed oil (which can be heated up to 420 degrees while retaining its nutrients) and avocado oil (can be heated up to 490 degrees while retaining its nutrients). Olive oil, like many other oils, is sensitive to heat and burn in seconds. Any oil that burns not only intoxicates the food but it also loses it properties such as vitamin E and Omega3 and 6.

- Instead of peanut butter (which causes allergic reactions in many people) try almond butter.

- Instead of refined salt made in labs with chemicals, use salt low in sodium.

- Instead of potato chips (high in saturated and trans-fats) have almonds, seeds, nuts, etc...

- Instead of white rice (high in starch and low in fiber and nutrients) use brown rice, millet, couscous, buckwheat, wild rice, etc...

- Instead of cow milk (difficult to digest) and yogurts high in sugars, try unsweetened soy and almond milk, plain yogurt, tofu, and kefir.

- Instead of mayonnaise (high in saturated fat and cholesterol) use "vegenaise" made from grape seed.

- Instead of commercial jam made with artificial flavors, use jam that does not have artificial flavors, colors, added sugars or the additive aspartame.

- Instead of always eating the same vegetables, rotate them and dare to try a new one every week. Try vegetables considered to have healing properties such as kohlrabi, bitter melon, celery roots, parsley root, kale, rutabaga, turnips, and parsnips among others.

- Instead of refined sugar (which weakens your immune system, dehydrates you and causes obesity) use stevia sugar and/or agave nectar.

FAKE FAT

SEVEN STEPS TO LOSE FAKE FAT

WHAT IS FAKE FAT?

According to nutrition, "fake fat" is only inflammation and water retention in the body as a result of an allergic reaction or hypersensitivity to some foods. You can lose up to 4 pounds of this fake fat in 1 week when you watch what you eat. Losing 4 to 5 pounds per week is not healthy unless what you are losing is fake fat. After ridding your body of the fake fat, you can continue to nourish your body by avoiding foods that cause allergic reactions. Then you will only lose 2 to 3 pounds per week. So, how do we get rid of "fake fat"?

Step #1: Temporarily avoid wheat, cereal and tortillas for at least 2 weeks. If you find you feel better when you don't eat them, just avoid it permanently. Replace flour or whole wheat bread, tortillas, cereals and pastas with sprouted flourless ones. Many people are sensitive to wheat because of the protein known as gluten and although it is important to eat fiber you can get it from sprouted grains, vegetables, fruits, and seeds.

Step #2: Temporarily avoid dairy products. If you are allergic to cow's milk, replace it with almond milk, plain yogurt, or kefir. It is best to eat yogurt and kefir before breakfast on an empty stomach. Kefir is related to yogurt and they are both high in calcium, digestive enzymes, and microorganisms that keep the balance of the internal eco-system of the body. Kefir is better because it has a type of probiotic or friendly micro-flora that is not found in yogurt, such as Lactobacillus Caucasus, Leuconostoc, Acetobacter Species, and

Streptococcus Species. It is also more nutritious and therapeutic than yogurt. Kefir has complete protein, essential minerals, and several types of essential vitamin B. The calcium in cow's milk can also be found in most vegetables, yogurt, kefir, and cottage cheese. Ghee butter has less saturated fat and fewer calories. This skimmed butter can be used moderately on your foods once they are already cooked. Margarine is not recommended because of its hydrogenated oil, which is dangerous for the heart.

Step #3: Eliminate refined sugars. (PG 104) Refined sugars must be eliminated permanently from your diet, but if you wish to use them do so sporadically. If you have candidiasis[1] eliminate all sugars for two weeks, including fresh and dry fruit, flours, vinegar, yeast, and all fermented products (except sprouted grain tortillas that do not have yeast or gluten). After cleaning your system entirely, add 1 fruit per day to your diet for the following 2 weeks. After those 2 weeks you can have 2 fruits per day for 2 months. Finish this cleansing and you can have your 3 servings of fruit per day once again.

NOTE: The only sugar substitute that you can use during this cleansing routine after the first 2 weeks is the plant sweetener stevia.

Step # 4: Try the water diet. Foods considered water foods are fruits, salads, vegetables and root juices, chamomile tea, rooibos, and green tea without sweetener. You can add a teaspoon of extra virgin cold-press olive oil, sea salt, lemon, and crushed garlic. This diet will give your digestive apparatus a break and it will help you digest your food better. If you have candidiasis you can also do this

---

1   Candidiasis symptoms include allergies, itchy skin, ulcers, psoriasis, fatigue, irritability, insomnia, yeast infections or fungus on the feet, fingernails, and toenails.

diet but you must avoid fruit. It is recommended you do this diet 1 day per week or simply have fruit, green vegetable juices and salads for breakfast for 15 days.

Step # 5: Don't drink a single drop of alcohol. Alcohol is a kind of sugar that has too many calories and if you don't burn them off, they soon become fat. Alcohol slows down your metabolism, oxidizes your cells, and dehydrates your organism—especially the colon—and it prematurely ages you.

Step # 6: Reduce your caloric intake by eating smaller portions. This will help you digest better and absorb more nutrients from the foods you eat. So, be careful not to think that just because you are eating healthy foods you can eat large portions.

Step # 7: Practice food rotation. Rotating foods not only helps you avoid getting bored from eating the same foods all of the time, but it also keeps you from developing allergic reactions, which cause organ and tissue inflammation and water retention.

SATURATED FAT VERSUS ESSENTIAL OILS

Why do we say that saturated fat is the main cause for obesity and is the most dangerous element to our health? The very simple reason is that the body does not recognize it as a natural fat and so does not digest it. This fat ends up sticking to the walls of our arteries, where it obstructs circulation and increases the risk of a heart attack or stroke. Saturated fats are those that come from red meat, fried foods, and hydrogenated foods such as margarine. Most foods commercially processed to become low-fat go through a hydrogenation process in which the liquid oils are transformed to solids.

So, despite the labels on the packaging, these so-called "low-fat" foods are in reality actually pretty high in trans-fat which is worse; not only because the body does not identify that fat as natural, but because now these foods have chemicals and additives. With all this they become artificial foods with no nutritional value. Continuous consumption of such food can lead to heart disease, cancer and chronic obesity.

IMPORTANT: Remember to use organic, fresh and live foods as much as possible. Canned foods can be used in emergencies, but even then you must pay attention to the labels and avoid foods high in saturated fats, sugars (especially corn syrup) and sodium. Foods high in trans-fats and saturated fats are: flan, ice cream, pastries, donuts, cookies, bagels, croissants, and most potato chips, fries, fried foods, red meat and all types of animal products, deli meats and meats cured with nitrates and nitrites.

TYPES OF FAT

Saturated fats, unsaturated, monounsaturated, poly-unsaturated and trans-fats.

Saturated Fats: These fats are considered bad because they dangerously increase your cholesterol levels and cause circulatory problems. They are found in animal products (meat, milk and their derivatives). The best way to identify saturated fat is to see if they become solid when chilled. Most plants do not have saturated fat except palm and coconut oils.

Unsaturated Fats: These fats are liquid at room temperature and are considered good fats because they can help keep cholesterol levels at normal levels, thereby helping to prevent heart disease.

Monounsaturated Fats: Fats that thicken when they are cooled but do not become solids, like peanut and olive oil.

Poly-unsaturated Fats: These fats stay liquid even when cold and we find them in fish oil, sunflower oil and soy oil.

Trans-fats: Liquid fats that after a process called hydrogenation become solids, these types of fats can be found in margarines, pastries and fries. Oil is heated and put under pressure for hours with nickel, hydrogen and carbon gas. The hydrogen and carbon atoms are what help the oil become creamy and solid. Then to finalize the process, this solidified, hydrogenated fat is then filtered and whitened with chemicals.

EATING SCHEDULE

If you work nights and sleep during the day you may ask yourself, how will I be able to eat well and lose weight? Perhaps your goal is to use nutrition to gain weight. Or, maybe you are simply trying to avoid illnesses.

If you have to work nights, it doesn't matter if it is 2:00 or 3:00pm when you wake up; you must begin your day with breakfast during the first hour, 2 hours later eat a snack, like plain yogurt and ½ of a fruit, eat lunch 2 hours later, eat dinner 3 hours later, have supper 4 hours later, you must eat supper 3 hours before laying down or going to bed. Ideally you should eat every 3 hours and make them small meals from all the groups like protein complex carbs and essential fatty acids.

Eat smaller portions of food, no matter what time you get up. For example, if your routine has you up at 5:00 am and work starts at 6:00 am, eat half of your breakfast at once, and then when you get your morning break, eat the other half.

If you're not too hungry during one of your breaks or lunch, eat a piece of fruit or salad and drink vegetable juice that you prepared at home. Don't forget to drink water, too. In other words, divide your breakfast and lunch in four parts. In between meals, add 2 snacks (fruits with almonds or vegetables) and again before going to sleep. It doesn't matter what time it is, just make sure your last snack or dinner is 3 hours before you go to bed.

If for whatever reason you can't eat at home or bring your own food, eat something healthy, grilled or steamed, etc... Avoid creamy dressings, white flours, fried foods, and refined sugars. Even fast food places (which I do not recommend) sell grilled chicken,

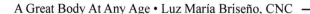

sandwiches, salads, and fruits.

And if you're going to eat something that is not healthy, do it without feeling guilty and enjoy it! Just make sure the serving size is small and you don't do it too often. Feeling guilty or worried after eating something on your "forbidden list" is not too healthy because these feelings acidify the organism and acid excess not only accumulates in the stomach in the form of fat, but also damages the arteries, joints, and main body organs.

JUICE DRINKS

GREEN JUICE FOR THE EYES

- 2 ounces of carrot
- 2 ounces of kale*
- 2 ounces of mustard greens*
- 2 ounces of turnips*

This juice is excellent for the sight and also for nocturnal blindness, to reinforce the immunological and digestive system.

*These vegetables can be found in most supermarkets that offer organic foods.

REJUVENATION JUICE

- 2 ounces of carrot
- 2 ounces of spinach
- 2 ounces of broccoli
- 2 ounces of parsley

This juice helps strengthen the immune system, improves anemia, prevents body cell oxidation, strengthens the brain and the nervous system, reduces bad cholesterol, prevents and improves diabetes, and if all that weren't enough, it also helps to form new collagen (collagen is a tissue protein; without this protein the skin prematurely wrinkles).

ENERGY JUICE

- 2 ounces of kale

- 2 ounces broccoli

- 2 ounces of spinach

- 2 ounces of turnip

This juice helps strengthen the immune system to restore muscle tissue. The anti-oxidants in these vegetables fight cancer cells, reverse premature aging, fight acne and skin problems, and improve sight (even night-blindness). They cure respiratory problems, help repair the digestive system, improve cardiovascular problems, strengthen the brain and nervous system, protect against viruses and bacteria, reduce cholesterol, prevent diabetes, increase energy, and diminish appetite caused by anxiety.

PRECAUTION: People with hypothyroidism must avoid raw cruciferous (broccoli, cauliflower, Brussels sprouts, cabbage, kale, turnips, collards, radish, rutabaga, and mustard greens). The chemistry in these vegetables changes when they are cooked so that the thyroid gland is stimulated to produce thyroxin—one of the metabolism hormones. If you suffer from hyperthyroidism, you should eat raw cruciferous to help decrease the excessive production of thyroxin.

SKIPPING MEALS

WHY SHOULD YOU NOT ONLY EAT ONCE A DAY?

When we only eat once a day we don't eat; rather, we devour our food. And not only that, but we do it fast without chewing thoroughly. In order to learn to read, write, draw, drive, etc..., we take the time to study carefully. Why is it that for something so important like maintaining out body in good condition, we do not take the time to learn to eat healthy? Well, it is never too late to start.

The stomach can only digest 400 calories in each meal for people who don't work out. In people who do work out, the body can digest 500 calories each meal. The rest of the non-digested calories consumed turn into fat, cellulite, and bacteria.

With that in mind, the risks of skipping meals include suffering from stomach illnesses, gastritis, constipation, ulcers, depression, obesity, diabetes, and many more unpleasant problems. The main reason people gain weight is not because they eat 3 times a day; not even because they have snacks between meals, but because they skip meals. Then, when they do eat, they consume food until they are extremely full and/or they eat any piece of junk food that may come to hand.

The stress caused by skipping meals combined with a hectic lifestyle, including emotional stress, nervousness, sadness, depression, irritability, fear, resentment, and poor nutrition, wears out the adrenal glands. These glands are in charge of releasing certain types of hormones (adrenaline and glucocorticoids) to fight stress. Obviously, the more we use these glands without nourishing them, the more health problems we have. Or, if we already have a disease, it worsens drastically.

High levels of adrenaline and cortisol in the blood destroy muscle tissue and acidify the blood. This acidification destroys cells, deteriorates the body defense system and causes all the above mentioned problems.

This type of nutritional stress also activates the defense mechanism, scaring the body due to the lack of food, and as consequence signals the body to retain fat.

RECOMMENDATIONS

Avoid: Fried foods, large animal protein portions, saturated fats, and processed foods because they have additives, chemicals, colorings, and artificial flavors and are too high in sodium and sugar. Drink 12 glasses of water per day. If you don't drink water you won't be able to remove the acidity from your body.

Alkalinize your organism: This means you have to clean your blood stream from the excess of acid with a healthy balanced diet high in green vegetables, a bit of fruit, some whole grains, seeds, and animal protein in moderate quantities.

Amongst the best supplements to alkalinize the blood are found in powdered green veggies. This supplement will help you control your appetite and restore your body's balance.

MAXIMUM DIGESTION

HOW TO ACHIEVE MAXIMUM DIGESTION

In order for foods to be digested to the maximum, protein (meats and dairy products) must be combined with some type of raw vegetable like lettuce, cucumber, jicama etc..., with Italian dressing or simply olive oil and lemon. The enzymes in raw vegetables not only help digestion but they also help make protein into amino acids to repair tissue and form new muscle.

If you have never eaten raw vegetables avoid raw cruciferous ones (which can cause intestinal inflammation). Instead, start by steam cooking them until you can gradually tolerate them raw.

Carbohydrates and starches (potatoes, legumes, tortillas, bread, cereal and pastas) must be combined with vegetables, non-saturated oil/fats like butter, virgin and raw olive oil, almond milk, nuts and seeds.

Fruit is a lot better if it is eaten alone and on an empty stomach. Unless you suffer from diabetes, it is better to eat them right after eating. If eaten alone, fruit helps detox the blood stream and allows the body to fully-absorb food nutrients.

Even though seeds and nuts are proteins they can be combined with carbs for the simple reason that they are natural proteins.

Bananas, dried fruits and avocados are the only fruits that are digested not only in the stomach, but also in the intestines. Other fruits only go through the stomach to later be digested through the intestines.

Drinking warm water with lemon 15 minutes before each meal, helps prepare the gastric juices for better digestion and absorption of nutrients.

Eating animal protein without carbs (vegetables) or vice versa can eventually cause glucose crashes and diabetes. The stomach produces chloric digestive acid strong enough to metabolize or decompose food. It is a myth that you should not eat protein with carbs or starches.

The secret to good digestion is in having moderate portions of each one of the food groups. You cannot eat large protein portions of any food without paying the price of bad digestion.

The body needs balance. A balanced diet has a bit of protein, a bit of carbs and a bit of fat. If you decide to eat brown rice or whole grain bread or sprouted grain bread, it must also be in small portions. It's best to alternate rice and potatoes than eating them together. Furthermore, you should eat no more than about a tennis ball-sized portion of them. As far as bread and tortillas go, the portion must be 1 slice of bread, 1 tortilla or 1/2 of a large tortilla.

NUTRITION FOR THE DISABLED

What happens to a disabled person's body when they eat junk food like hot dogs, sodas, potato chips, French fries, hamburgers, cookies, pastries, nachos with cheese, doughnuts, bagels, coffee, wheat bread, alcohol, cigarettes, ice cream, crackers and chocolate chip cookies etc...?

These kinds of junk food take 10 years away from the life of this person. Not only that, but junk food opens the door for deadly diseases. Worst of all, throughout this unnecessarily-shortened life, the disabled person must endure an excess of physical pain, irritability, depression, resentment and even hatred.

FOODS WITH MEGAHERTZ

You must remember that the body generates energy in the form of electricity. So, the food we consume is also measured in energy. There are foods positive with megahertz (MHZ) that give you energy and others are negative that take it from you. For example, some processed foods with chemicals, additives, and preservatives and with artificial flavors and colors have 0 MHZ, while others have negative MHZ. By contrast, fresh foods like tomatoes, onions, garlic, etc..., have between 15 and 22 MHZ. Fish, cucumbers and almonds have approximately 320 MHZ. A piece of cake with ice cream has about negative 400 MHZ. In other words, because these megahertz are negative, they rob your body all the electricity which is the energy taken from the body's nutrients.

What does healthy food do to the body of an incapacitated person?

A healthy diet may not change the genetic structure with which they were born and it might not restore their memory or strength to the point where they can walk again but at least it will not take years of his/her life. It will prevent new diseases and more importantly it will keep him/her happy without suffering, without physical pain and without depression. That is what nutrition does to the body of a disabled or ill person.

Since hot dog buns are made of refined flour it does not have any fiber or nutrients. As soon as you eat white bread it becomes sugar and if you do not burn it off with exercise it becomes fat that deposits itself in the liver and in all the fat storages in the body and if there are no other spaces available it forms new fat cells.

Hot dog sausages are made with garbage or the fat and meat leftovers that are not sold or cannot be sent out to meat markets or grocery stores. Those leftovers are grinded with tasty artificial flavorings and voila the sausages taste great. The small amount of protein that it might have is lost with the added preservatives and artificial flavors. All of those chemical are toxic that feed the cancer cells in the body.

Ketchup or tomato sauce has more artificial sugar than anything else; it is basically chemicals with sugar. Some of its ingredients are: vinegar, sugar, salt, and spices with clove artificial flavorings, cinnamon, onion and celery.

MUSCLES

WHY DOES YOUR BODY EAT ITS OWN MUSCLE TISSUE?

In a balanced diet we eat animal protein, carbs and fats, but since there are different types of protein with carbs and fats, we must specify the difference between these foods. If animal protein is eaten in small portions, the body does not have a problem metabolizing it and using it to repair tissue. Even though vegetable protein has some amino acids it is more difficult to find the perfect combination of essential amino acids to repair tissue in these foods. Refined carbs from refined flours and simple sugar are very different than complex carbs in veggies and sprouted grains.

Complex carbs are high on fiber, vitamins and minerals, but refined carbs have had the fiber removed. That is precisely where we find the nutrients! The body needs essential fatty acids that act like lubricants for the main body organs and skin. These can be found in foods such as seeds, vegetable oils and avocados. Meanwhile, the body does not recognize hydrogenated oils made into solids, so it does not use them at all. It only processes them and stores them in saturated fat form.

Many people know they abuse starches, but since half of their caloric intake should come from carbs on the same plate, they eat just the protein and fat in the mistaken belief that they are getting the right carbs. For example, they serve themselves a plate with the following portions; half pasta, one fourth chicken and one fourth has salad with olive oil. From the moment the pasta reaches the mouth, digestion begins by turning it into simple sugar. The body can store a small amount of sugar in glycogen form in the muscles and in the liver. The remainder that cannot be stored in glycogen form is used as fuel for immediate energy, but cells can only burn simple sugar in small amounts. So, what happens to the rest of the simple sugars that we ate from that pasta plate?

What happens is that it becomes fat! What happens to the protein and fat in the oils that you ate? That becomes fat, too! Part of that protein you took from your plate and ate will be used to repair and maintain muscle but again, the cells only use small amounts at a time. The rest becomes sugar to be stored in saturated fat form. When the body uses the sugar stored in glycogen form for fuel, all that extra fat gets stuck; the cells do not use saturated fat when there is sugar or glycogen available.

WHY ARE PROTEIN AND FAT NOT USED FOR FUEL?

The body first has to use up the glycogen and the simple sugar or glucose in the body before going to the fat storages. If you eat fat and sugar at the same time, your body will burn the sugar before it starts using up the fat, but if you eat a bit of sugar and a bit of fat and your body burns the sugar and then still needs fuel for energy, it will first go to the glycogen storages before burning the fat that you just ate. If you are used to eating sugars and starches often, your body will get used to burning sugar from any part of the body (including the sugar or glucose in the muscles) before using up the fat as a source of fuel.

When you are young, your metabolism is more flexible. It can change fuel sources rather easily, but the older you get, the more your cells get used to your individual routine of eating and your body adjusts accordingly on a regular basis and as a matter of habit. If, when you were young your body got used to burning mostly sugar, your metabolism will habitually look for sugar to burn when you are old.

If your body has habitually learned to become a sugar burning machine over the years of your life, be careful! Your cells may have become addicted to sugar will kick you into sugar cravings without caring where that sugar comes from. If you go to sleep while still in a sugar burning stage, your body will still look for it to continue burning sugar even while you sleep.

Day or night, whenever your cells are hungry they immediately look for sugar in the starchy glycogen of the liver and muscle storages, even if the body would rather store this type of sugar or glycogen for emergencies like when you have to flee from danger.

IT IS DANGEROUS TO USE MUSCLE FOR FUEL

If your cells are addicted to burning sugar, they will find a way to metabolize the muscle protein and even bone protein to turn them into sugar. This is more dangerous than you can possibly imagine! This destructive process causes osteoporosis faster than not taking calcium supplements, and even if you do resistance exercises, your muscles will not experience good results.

As long as there is sugar in your system, your metabolism hormones give the order to burn it rather than fat—even if you have many extra fat pounds to spare. Cells hungry for sugar will only pass by fat storages without touching any of it. So, if you follow a diet high in carbs and sugars or high in protein, your body will continue its habit of burning sugar and storing fat instead of attacking the fat.

As long as you are resistant to the hunger hormone leptin, you'll continue being hungry because your brain has lost the ability to listen to this hormone. It is believed that when fat storages increase, the body releases leptin to the bloodstream. This is basically a signal to the hypothalamus (part of the nervous system) that there is enough food in the stomach and that the hunger should subside.

To be resistant to this hormone makes your brain order your body to store and retain fat. As a consequence, all your body will burn and metabolize its sugar.

HOW TO BREAK THE ADDICTION OF FEEDING FROM YOUR MUSCLES

In order to break the vicious cycle of habitual sugar-burning and the addiction of your cells to burn sugar, you will need to reprogram your brain and order the cells to burn fat for fuel instead. When this happens, your cells metabolize fat even if you're not eating.

Whenever your cells need energy they will get it from your fat storages—even while you're sleeping, and best of all, your body will not be robbing your muscles or bones in search of sugar. Your brain will not care if it gets the fat from what you just ate, or from the fat stored in your waist or hips.

At the same time, the arteries in your body will be able to burn their own fat. You will feel satisfied and will not be as hungry, since the cells will be constantly feeding themselves from fat you've already stored.

THE SECRET TO BURNING FAT AS FUEL

The secret to stop burning more sugar than fat is in eating fewer grains, less starches and no gluten. Instead, eat sprouted grains in small portions.

Avoid refined sugars and white flours regulate fruit consumption and eat more essential fatty acids. Remember that what you eat most is what you burn most.

If you eat more sugars you will burn more sugars and your brain will ask for more sugars.

Eat less protein. If you eat too much protein, the excess becomes sugar and you burn sugar.

If you eat saturated fats, its excess is stored as saturated fat, so watch your intake of this kind of fat.

If you eat more foods high in essential fatty acids as part of a balanced diet you will burn additional fat.

Avoid or restrict foods that become sugar and then fat; bleached and brown flours, grains (except sprouted grains), starches including potatoes, bananas and vegetables or fruits with no fiber.

Foods that burn fat: Vegetables with fiber and no starch, fish, chicken, and lean meats, seeds, nuts, avocado, cabbage, citrus fruits especially lemon and olive, flax and grape seed oils.

NOTE: Sweet and citric fruits except lemon should be consumed during the day—preferably not after 5 or 6 p.m. These will tend to cause an allergic reaction.

BASIC NUTRITION

These are the basic points in nutrition, which if you truly follow them will give you immediate results. If you have a serious health condition check with your doctor first and at the same tame watch what you eat. Remember: you have to be patient with your body and take care of it in order to see the benefits of nutrition. For every year you did not take care of your organism you need at least 6 weeks of real nutrition in order to repair the damages.

A nutritious diet is one in which you must avoid and/or entirely eliminate foods such as bleached flours and refined sugars, lake pastries, chips, cookies, chocolates, coffee, soda, alcohol, cigarettes, fried foods. Do not skip meals. Instead, eat quality meals every 3 hours in small portions.

Modern processed and refined foods are poison for the body. As long as you continue to ingest these poisons, you will not be able to improve your health or lose weight. Even if your goal is to gain weight you won't be able to achieve that either. If you have a fast metabolism that makes it tough for you to gain weight, fast food will only make your metabolism faster and weight gain will be that much harder.

Eat sprouted grain bread, but if you are allergic to gluten or sick, use flourless sprouted bread cereal and tortillas. You can find them in the supermarkets that carry healthy, organic foods. Also include brown rice, chicken breast, white fish, salmon, turkey, salads with lettuce and raw veggies and olive or grape seed oils and sea salt, chicken or fish soup, 2 fruits per day and 3 or 4 raw vegetables. Don't forget you also need to drink 2 or 3 liters of water per day. Eat 5 or 6 time per day: breakfast, snack, lunch, snack, and dinner. Also, if you go to sleep late and you get hungry, have another protein snack—no carbs.

DON'T FORGET TO BRING SNACKS: Whenever you go on a trip, always carry snacks like almonds, fruit, cheese, raw veggies and toast. A snack is always better than an empty stomach. If it is hard for you to lose weight, eat flourless sprouted tortilla, bread or cereal only once per day.

BREAKFAST: It is very important that breakfast be a light but nutritious meal. Breakfast turns on your metabolism so that you can absorb vitamins and minerals better throughout the day. Make a regular habit out of eating a nutritious breakfast and you'll find your health drastically improved, while at the same time you will lose or gain weight quickly, whichever may be your need. If you are not over- or under-weight, you will maintain your ideal weight while preventing degenerative diseases.

FOODS THAT ARE HARMFUL TO PEOPLE THAT ARE SICK

People who are ill need more alkaline than acidic foods, so the following items should be avoided during illness: citric fruits (except lemon), dairy products (except kefir and plain yogurt), chocolate, coffee, fried foods, red meats, processed foods, sugar, wheat, yeast, vinegar, and dry grains. Convalescent diets including grains require that you soak any grain for 14 hours then toss the water and rinse the grains before cooking them because this process removes acidity.

VEGETABLES YOU SHOULD AVOID IF YOU HAVE ARTHRITIS

The fruits and vegetables that people with any sort of arthritis should avoid are; potatoes, eggplant, tomatoes, and nightshade vegetables and green bell peppers (you can eat red, yellow, and orange bell peppers). After avoiding these for 6 weeks, you can eat them once or twice per week and rotate them, 1 vegetable at a time and making sure that it is ripe.

FOODS DIABETICS SHOULD AVOID

Diabetics should make sure they avoid refined sugar, brown sugar and all kinds of simple sugars such as honey or molasses. Cooked carrots and parsnips should also be left out of a diabetic diet; these vegetables must be eaten raw in a juice or shredded on a salad so that they will help reduce alcohol and sugar cravings. Diabetics should also avoid sports drinks, carbonated drinks, cereals, corn tortillas, millet, wheat, bleached flour, dried fruit, commercial fruit juices, white rice, oven-baked and fried potatoes (though boiled potatoes are ok).

SALSA TO PREVENT OXIDATION OF CELLS

Antioxidant Salsa

- 1/2 cup of parsley

- 3 cilantro stems

- 1 fresh oregano stem

- 1/2 of an onion

- 3 fresh garlic cloves

- sea salt to taste

- 5 tablespoons of extra-virgin cold-press olive oil

- the juice of 1 medium lemon

- 2 fresh jalapeños (not pickled)

If you do not have arthritis you may add 1 raw tomato and ½ of a red, yellow and orange bell pepper.

Grind everything in a food processor and store in the refrigerator. This salsa can be used as a side for any dish or to make guacamole and if you don't have any health problems you can also mix it with the traditional *chile de molcajete* (salsa ground on a mortar stone).

SMOOTHIES:

Make your own anti-oxidant smoothies by mixing:

- Almond milk, 1% skim milk, plain yogurt or kefir

- 2 dates or any fresh or frozen fruit (strawberries, raspberries, mango, etc...)

- 1 packet of stevia sweetener

- 1 or 2 tablespoons of mixed ground seeds (sunflower, sesame, flax and pumpkin seeds)

IMPORTANT: Make sure that you sweat 3 times per week doing some sort of exercise or physical activity. Once you break a sweat continue working out for 15 or 20 minutes more. Breaking a sweat is a sign that your body is changing fuel sources and that it is now using fat as a source of energy.

NUTRITION FOR BEGINNERS

1. Reduce refined salt consumption and replace it with sea salt and fresh herbs. You can grow a little herb garden on your kitchen window sill to add more flavor to your dishes and diminish the use of refined salt.

2. Don't have temptations handy; just don't have any junk food in your house. Any time you have anxiety attacks and cravings for cookies, chips, candies or any other junk food, drink an 8 ounce glass of water with lemon and wait 5 to 10 minutes. Many times thirst is confused with hunger. Then if you are still hungry or have cravings, eat 1/2 of a fruit and 6 almonds.

3. Cook all of your soups including chicken and beef so that they can cool off and you can remove the excess fat that settles on the top.

4. At the restaurant ask for a doggie bag. Separate a half portion of the food before you start eating, and put it in your take-home container.

5. If you have never eaten vegetables or are not used to eating them frequently, simply add them to your favorite foods. For example add veggies to your sandwich and serve your rice and meat dishes with vegetables and a salad. If you like stuffed peppers serve them with a green salad and steamed vegetables.

6. An easy way to identify foods with trans-fats is by paying attention to words on food labels such as grated cheese, *parmigiana* (parmesan cheese), tempura, alfredo creamy, *carbonara*, etc... Consume foods with these things in them only once in a while and in small portions.

7. Stop whatever else you are doing when it is time to eat. Avoid driving or talking on the phone, texting, worrying, fighting, walking, cooking, and doing your make-up, etc... while you eat your food. When you eat and do something else at the same time, you do not pay attention to what you are eating or the way you are doing it. That is how you end up eating faster and more than you should. Eating quickly under pressure and/or when you are distracted causes intestinal spasms, indigestion, inflammation, gases and abdominal pain.

8. Leave something on you plate every time you eat. You don't have to throw it away; just save it for later when you get hungry again. Try and see if you get full with 3/4 of what you are used to eating. Remember that it takes the brain 20 minutes to get the signal from the satisfied hormone (leptin), which tells the stomach it is full. So, have a salad with olive oil and a snack with essential fatty acids because these activate leptin. Eat slowly and eat smaller portions.

9. Remember that some people need more food than others. Start by knowing what your own need is and the portions you need from every food group. For example, did you know that one brown rice serving should be the size of a tennis ball and that a serving of meat should be the size of the palm of your hand and as thick as a deck of cards?

10. Try something different than what you are used to and you might discover that you like healthy food more than you thought.

11. Find a substitute that you may enjoy. For example, try skimmed milk or almond milk for your shakes instead of whole milk. Swap white bread for flourless sprouted grain bread.

12. Take your lunch to work. Not only will you eat truly fresh and healthy foods, but you will also save a fortune.

13. Enjoy dessert without feeling guilty. Use portion-control when eating them occasionally now and then. This way you will do

well.

14. Tell your mother-in-law (nicely, of course) to stop putting more food on your plate than you will be able to eat.

15. Ask your partner not to give you chocolates or sweets on holidays. Instead, ask him to get you perfume, a flower, or maybe something different like a diamond, a car or a gold bar.

16. Make changes gradually but consistently over time and be patient; remember that you did not get sick and gain weight overnight. In the same manner, allow your body to heal itself gradually so that you do not become frustrated. For every year that you were careless with your organism you will need to take care of it for 6 weeks since body cells are regenerated every 6 weeks. Eat smart and healthy, and do not let an event interrupt that program.

For example, my son Mateo grew up on junk food because his mom (the author of this book) did not know anything about nutrition and like many of you thought that restaurants could not possibly serve foods that were bad for people!

So let us see how long it would take Mateo to compensate for the years of bad nutrition.

If for every year of poor nutrition in the past the body needs 6 weeks of good nutrition in the present and Mateo is 21 years old, let's multiply 6 weeks by 21. This gives Mateo 126 weeks or 2.6 years of good nutrition before he would be able to overcome the effects of his years eating a poor diet.

CHEMICALS

Pesticides, fungicides, herbicides and chemical preservatives present in most foods not only sicken your liver and blow you up like a balloon but also cause deadly cancers. Industrial and agricultural chemicals contaminate the earth, water and our food. Did you know that Los Angeles is the city with the most contaminated air in the U.S.? New Orleans is in the list of cities with the highest contamination of water. Cities like these also have populations with the most serious cases of diseases like rhinitis, bronchitis, asthma, migraines, allergies and irritability.

Our body has the ability to repair and eliminate abnormal cells, but when our defense system or our immune system is chronically tired or slow, how is our body going to get rid of all those abnormal cells? It won't be able to do that, and these abnormal cells will keep accumulating in the tissues of different organs.

What do you think all those chemicals in pre-packaged foods filled with additives and artificial flavors like hot dogs and chips with cheese, fried flours, chocolate chip cookies, potato chips, saturated fats, etc..., do to your body? Besides the immediate damage these modern, synthetic types of foods do on their own, imagine the damage they can do if consumed daily and in large quantities.

By eating these kinds of foods you are mistreating your body. Such foods kill the body gradually by weakening the immune system and then eventually causing chronic inflammation, fat deposits, malignant tumors and the birth of new cells that become cancer.

Did you know that there are some synthetic foods that don't have a single natural flavor particle in them? In fact, there are foods made up entirely of chemicals like gum, breath mints, coffee creamers, sugar substitutes, candies, etc... Why do you suppose the food industry uses chemicals rather than natural products? Check out the 5 main reasons listed here:

1. The food industry uses chemicals rather than natural ingredients so that their product does not spoil on the grocery shelves so they do not lose a single cent. Those chemical preservatives assure their profit is safe even after years and even if the food is almost all synthetic.

2. The food industry uses more chemicals than natural ingredients because these ingredients are available year-round even if it is not their season. This appeals to people who want everything ready to eat even if it is in a can, jar or box; immediately ready to heat or defrost.

3. The food industry uses more chemicals than natural foods in order to add vitamins and minerals to foods that have lost most of their minerals and vitamins during the process of preparation. That is why you see so many cereals enriched with vitamins and minerals or milk enriched with vitamin D, etc... The problem is that these vitamins are not recognized as such by the body. On the contrary, all that these food enrichments do is dirty the blood.

4. The food industry uses more chemicals than natural foods so that food tastes good. If you have ever lived in Mexico you might remember the *Sabritas* chips billboards that said "I bet you cannot eat just one". Chemicals have the purpose of making you addicted to their product. There are special chemicals made to make your body need them so that you can become addicted to that food.

5. The last reason why the food industry benefits from using chemicals rather than natural products is so that the food looks more appealing so that you will buy it. It is impossible to list all the ways this is done, but for the moment let's just say that meat is injected with nitrates and nitrites so that it will

look fresh and it has a little color in the package; these products will cause cancer with long term use. Lettuce, vegetables and fruits also get chemical treatments so that they will look fresh, green or whatever their natural color in the produce section of the market.

INTERNAL REPAIR AND CLEANSING

When you have liver problems it hardly ever hurts unless there is inflammation. The liver of a "modern" person is generally tired and in poor condition due to excess ingestion of processed products with so many chemicals, due to the lack of drinking water and also due to unhealthy eating. The formation of blood is precisely one the livers main responsibilities.

The stomach, small intestine, salivary and gastric glands, pancreas and liver form part of the digestive apparatus. The liver is not only a filter between the heart and the intestines it is also a biliary organ and an endocrine gland. That is to say, the liver is one of the most important organs in the body—almost as important as the heart or the brain.

LET YOUR LIVER AND DIGESTIVE SYSTEM REST

For 2 or 3 days, every food you eat you should put it in a blender. This will allow your digestive apparatus to rest so that your tired liver can recover quickly. Vegetable juices with a bit of fruit help detox the liver, especially if every Monday you only drink juices, green salads with raw shredded vegetables, lemon, olive oil, sea salt, fresh garlic and some organic fruit.

JUICES FOR LIVER DETOXIFICATION

Make juices with vegetables like cucumbers, green zucchini, sprouted alfalfa, all types of bean sprouts, cabbage, grapes, pears, carrots, kale, beats, ripe tomatoes (but not if you have arthritis), parsley, celery, and the juice of 2 lemons. Drink this juice 2 to 3 times per week and only eat easy to digest foods like salads and veggies. Vary and rotate the veggies so that you can take advantage of all the nutrients and also so that you don't get tired of the same tastes. You can do this kind of cleansing 1 time per week or 3 consecutive days per month. If you opt to do the monthly cleanse program, you can add blended chicken soup with chicken breast or fish soup and veggies only.

As soon as you wake up you should drink a glass of warm water with 1/2 of a lemon. Every time you get hungry, drink a glass of water and then a glass of juice. You can do this kind of cleanse for up to 7 days without any risks unless you are pregnant, lactating or if your doctor prohibits it.

WHEAT GRASS

Drink 1 ounce of wheat grass juice once a day for a week and then increase it to 2 ounces per day. This juice cleans the liver and prevents the growth of cancerous cells. Make sure you use the proper wheat grass juice-extractor.

ACCELERATING THE REPAIR OF EVERY ORGAN

Grind each of the following separately and in even portions:

- flax seeds

- sesame seeds

- sunflower seeds

- pumpkin seeds

Store this mixture in a container with a lid. You and all your family should take 1 tablespoon of it twice a day with water or green vegetables juices or MSM in powder or liquid form, the juice of 1 lemon, 1 teaspoon of wheat germ and 1 teaspoon of granulated lecithin. This drink will help you improve any health problem you may have a lot faster; mitigating any condition from digestive, muscle, nervous, cardiovascular and even immune and bone problems.

IMMUNE TEA FOR FLU AND COLD

Drink an immune tea to strengthen your immune system at the first sign of physical discomfort. When you feel stress is giving you a cold, cough or problems with your respiratory system, take the following tea infusion:

- 1 purple onion

- 5 garlic cloves

- 1 cinnamon stick

- Fresh or dried rosemary: whatever you can pinch with 3 fingers

Boil everything in 2 cups of water. As soon as it begins to boil, turn it off and cover it to sit for 30 to 60 minutes. Remove the cinnamon and rosemary and blend thoroughly so that you don't have to strain it (though you may do so if you wish). Serve it with the juice of 1 lemon; drink it 1 cup at a time several times a day until you finish it.

NOTE: This drink does not store well in the refrigerator. Whatever you do not drink in a 24 hour period you must discard. If your flu or cold is very strong you must do this for several days.

Infants as young as 6 months, kids of all ages, adults, elderly people, pregnant and lactating women can all drink this infusion. If your cold or flu does not include a cough you can add manuka honey to the immune tea infusion. You can find manuka honey at health food stores.

If your problem is a dry cough without any other symptoms perhaps what you have is acid reflux.

GAINING WEIGHT THROUGH NUTRITION

Gaining weight with nutrition is the opposite of losing weight without eating junk food. If you want to gain weight you must balance your metabolic system. You also have to increase your caloric intake and carefully select the sources of these calories.

When an obese or thin person eats a lot and does not feel full, it is because the body is hungry for nutrients. Even for a person who eats healthy and is still hungry, it is likely that he or she is not absorbing nutrients from foods due to any or all of the following conditions:

- excessive toxins

- high acid levels in the body

- physical or psychological health problems

- too much stress

Just like obesity, the lack of weight or being extremely thin is influenced by:

- poor nutrition since childhood or adolescence

- unleveled nutrients

- too much stress

You also may be extremely thin due to genetics (a naturally-fast metabolism) or because of your lifestyle. Let's remember that poor eating habits are also inherited and become a lifestyle.

If you are naturally thin and don't eat well, you will only get thinner. If you are naturally chubby and don't eat well, you will just go on gaining weight. Many people think that because they eat junk food and don't gain weight it is not harmful, but they are wrong. The chemicals and additives in prepackaged foods harm everyone. There are thin people with more illnesses than overweight people. This does not mean that it is right to be obese, but obesity is precisely a disease that the body uses to let you know you are not eating well. However, if your body does not give you any signs, as may be the case if you are too thin, what do you think happens? A serious disease eventually appears which has been growing silently for a long time and many times that disease turns out to be cancer.

It is harder for a thin person to gain weight when he or she is abusing processed toxic foods, junk food, prepackaged modern foods with chemicals and additives that cause addiction, and who also abuse coffee, cigarettes, alcohol, and other stimulants. For example, when an obese person has high acid levels, the body sends the acid to less dangerous places like fat cells. This happens so that the acid doesn't harm other vital organs, such as the liver, kidney, or heart.

If an obese person does not detox and regulate the levels of acid in the body, even if he or she eats healthy, he or she will not lose weight.

Now, imagine a person who is too thin and genetically can't store fat. Where do you think the body is going to send the excess acid toxins from junk food in an underweight individual? Extreme underweight is a chronic condition. There will come a time when alkaline reserves in the body run out. When this happens, excess acid goes right into joints and other deficient areas in the body.

A person acidifies their organism through any of the following ways:

- Angry thoughts

- Frustration

- Resentment

- Stress

- Lack of exercise and rest

- Lack of water

- Excess junk food

- Excess toxins from fried foods

- Excess animal protein and dairy products

- Lack of alkaline foods like green vegetables, salads, fruits etc...

- Cigarette and alcohol consumption

- Coffee, soda, refined sugar and bleached flours excess

- Lack of fiber

Coffee and cigarette combination generate nervous energy and frenetic mental activity that many people like to feel because it helps them function temporarily at work. Sadly though, it does not help them improve their health. Extremely thin people who have a hard time gaining weight need a combination of psychological therapy and counseling to manage stress... and—most important— good nutrition.

Stress can be reduced with physical exercise, relaxation and meditation to help your nervous system relax. Learning how to relax will help your metabolism. Then, if you also detox, your acid levels will balance off and with it your body will become rebalanced as well. Remember that a balanced body can absorb nutrients from foods and reduce acid more easily. If you want to gain weight consider the following tips:

- Add 500 calories of healthy foods to your diet per day or drink a protein shake once a day to gain 1 pound per week.

- Eat larger portions of food several times a day and healthy snacks between meals.

- Eat good portions of plain yogurt, cheese, nuts, almonds, avocado, brown rice, boiled or baked potatoes, whole wheat bread or sprouted grain bread with butter, soy or almond milk and shakes with fruits and yogurt. Do not eat just before going to bed because it may give you insomnia.

- Underweight people tend to feel cold, have poor circulation, fatigue and anemia. That is why fish from the sea is recommended especially for this condition. Olive oil on salads, red meat, poultry and liver contain protein to improve anything from anemia to fatigue, poor circulation and cold.

- Don't drink water before eating because this will take your appetite away. Drink it between meals only.

- Don't eat refined sugars because they are addictive and adversely affect your immune and metabolic system.

- Don't do high-impact aerobic exercise; it is better to walk, lift weights, and do yoga, Pilates, or any other resistance exercise.

PROTEIN SHAKE FOR WEIGHT GAIN

- ½ cup of unflavored soymilk or almond milk

- ½ cup of skimmed plain yogurt (low fat)

- 1 scoop (20 grams) of whey protein powder

- ½ cup of frozen berries (any type of fruit)

- 5 almonds

- 2 tablespoons of raw natural oats

*Protein powders are not recommended for children under 18 years of age.

Mix it in a blender until you achieve the desired consistency by adding more water or soymilk.

WEIGHT GAIN SUPPLEMENTS

Your multivitamins should contain:

-	Beta-carotene	20,000mg
-	Pantothenic Acid B	5,100mg
-	Cobalamin B12	50mg
-	Vitamin C (acerola)	500 to 3,000mg
-	Chromium	200mg
-	Magnesium	300 to 500mg
-	Manganese	5 to 10mg

- Selenium   200mg

- Molybdenum   200mg

- Silicone   50mg

Also:

- 1 multi amino acid, preferably sublingual cap liquid before each meal

- 2 tablespoons of flaxseed oil per day

- 1 capsule of digestive enzymes (bromelain) with each meal

- 1 tablespoon wheat germ

- 1 tablespoon granulated lecithin after each meal

- 1000mg Omega3 (fish oil) after every meal (men and women)

WARNING: On the days you do not drink your protein drink to gain weight you can take the multi-amino acids.

NOTE: If you have anemia (only if a doctor diagnoses you with moderate anemia) take liquid iron "flora vital" for one or two months and check your iron levels again.

SUPPLEMENTS

WHY IS IT SO IMPORTANT TO TAKE VITAMINS AND MINERALS IN FORM OF A SUPPLEMENT?

If all foods like fruits, vegetables, grains, seeds, and animal proteins didn't have fertilizers, chemicals, and hormones in them, our food would have more nutrients.

If fruits, vegetables, and grains were cut when they were ripe instead of harvested while they are still green, we would benefit more from the minerals of the earth. These foods take 10 days to get to the supermarkets once they are harvested and meat takes almost 2 weeks to get to the meat market after having sacrificed the animal.

If the soil where our food is grown would be left to rest, it would recover all of the necessary minerals for foods to have complete vitamins and minerals.

If we cooked food with a low flame, and we would eat vegetables semi-raw, we wouldn't rob part of its vitamins and minerals.

If we never fried foods at high temperatures, we would not add toxins into our systems.

If the foods we consume were not processed they wouldn't lose such insane amounts of minerals.

SUPPLEMENT DOSES FOR CHILDREN AND TEENAGERS

Adolescents from 13 to 17 years age:

¾ of the adult dose

Kids aged 7 to 12 years of age:

½ of an adult dose

Kids under 6 years of age:

¼ of an adult dose

RECOMMENDATION: Vitamins and supplements must be approved by a doctor for children less than 18 years of age, but it is more important for your children to have a good diet, water, exercise, vitamin and minerals with the appropriate doses for their ages.

VITAMINS

Here is quick guide to essential vitamins, minerals, anti-oxidants and amino acids:

- Vitamin A (beta carotene)

- Vitamin B1 & B2 (riboflavin)

- Vitamin B6 (pyridoxine)

- Vitamin B12 (cobalamin)

- Vitamin B3 (niacin)

- Panthothenic Acid, Biotin, Folic Acid, Inositol, Choline

- PABA (para aminobenzoic acid)

- Vitamin C (ascorbic acid)

- Vitamin D & Vitamin E

Vitamins and minerals are the micronutrients opposite to fat, protein, carbs that are also known as macronutrients found only in organic live foods like plants and animals. The chemistry of an animal's organism can make incomplete nutrients into protein, something the human body cannot do despite being so similar. That is why we need to supplement our bodies with nutritious foods and vitamins made from whole foods. Vitamin supplements will never replace the nutrients from live foods like lean meat, vegetable, fruits, and whole grain bread.

Still, taking vitamins and not eating well is like throwing money in the trash. For example, all types of Vitamin B can only be processed by the body if you take it right after eating protein and carbs, especially in the morning and afternoon. This helps regulate your glucose levels to give you energy throughout the day, especially if your job is stressful and you're used to drinking coffee and alcohol. It also helps you avoid sudden anxiety attacks and cravings for sugars and refined flours leading to obesity and diabetes.

VITAMINS AND MINERALS

Vitamins and minerals are the micronutrients opposite to fat, protein, carbs that are also known as macronutrients.

The formation of bone and the production of red cells are not possible without phosphorous, which can be found in meat, fish, and whole grains.

IRON: Iron is a hemoglobin constituent that carries oxygen to the blood stream.

Vitamins are essential to help the body release the energy from food nutrients so that our body functions properly and with that, are able to balance our hormone levels and strengthen the immune system. Vitamins also strengthen skin and tissue, protect arteries and especially help the brain to function properly.

VITAMINS CAN BE DIVIDED INTO TWO CATEGORIES: Water-soluble vitamins which must be replenished on a daily basis, and fat-soluble vitamins, which can be stored in large quantities.

Vitamin A (beta carotene)

Maximum dose of Vitamin A for women is 5,000 IU; for men 1,000 IU. Vitamin A overdose through supplements can cause intoxication. However, large quantities of vitamin A through food are handled by the body by absorbing what it needs and discarding what it does not through urine. Only in special circumstances will a doctor recommend you take 25,000 IU of vitamin A for 6 weeks for certain problems you may have, otherwise take the basic amount. Pregnant women should not use any type of liver because of its high content of Vitamin A).

Vitamin A:

- helps repair and build tissue

- keeps the skin looking young

- protects the mucus membranes in the mouth, nose and lungs from infections

- counter-attacks night-blindness to improves night-vision

- reverses premature aging

- helps heal skin problems, including acne, psoriasis and skin infections

- helps bone and teeth formation

- improves the respiratory, digestive, urinary and immune systems

Foods high in Vitamin A are: carrots, mangoes, oranges, papaya, peaches, liver and all fruits orange in color. These foods reduce the risk of getting lung and some oral cancers.

The symptoms of lack of Vitamin A include: poor vision, susceptibility to infections, shabby skin, lack of appetite, frequent fatigue, dental and gum problems and growth problems in infants and children.

Vitamin B1 (thymine)

- generates energy

- digests carbs

- helps the nervous system work properly

- strengthens the heart and stabilizes the appetite

- helps tone and grow muscle

Symptoms of Vitamin B1 deficiency include: lack of appetite, tiredness, irritability, insomnia, depression, constipation, gastrointestinal problems and heart trouble.

Vitamin B2 (riboflavin)

- helps metabolize carbs, fat and protein

- assists in building antibodies and red blood cells

- provides oxygen to cells

- maintains vision, skin, nails and hair in good condition

Symptoms of B2 deficiency include: itchiness around the eyes, dermatitis, digestive problems, oily skin and slow growth in children.

Vitamin B3 (niacin)

- improves blood circulation

- reduces cholesterol levels

- helps metabolize protein, fats and sugars

- lowers blood pressure

- helps distribute foods

- improves skin and the digestive system

Symptoms of Vitamin B3 deficiency include: premature aging, gastrointestinal problems, headaches, depression, and irritability, loss of appetite, insomnia, bad breath, mouth ulcers, diarrhea, nausea, dizziness, vomiting, memory loss, blurry vision, light sensibility and even schizophrenia.

Foods high in Vitamin B3 include liver, poultry, fish, meat, peanuts, whole grains, eggs and milk, and water soluble vitamins.

Vitamin B5 (pantothenic acid)

- helps gain energy from carbs, fats and proteins

- aids absorption of other vitamins

- helps the body resist stress

- assists in the formation of new cells

- improves functions of the central nervous system function

- helps the adrenal glands conserve energy in the body

- builds chemical neurotransmitters in charge of sending movement messages from one nerve to the next

- stimulates production of sex hormones

- fights infections when it creates antibodies

Symptoms of Vitamin B5 deficiency include: pain and burning sensation in the feet, abnormal feet, delayed growth, digestive problems, muscle cramps and stomach pains, stress, mental and physical fatigue, difficulty with concentration and irritability.

Foods high in Vitamin B5 are; peanuts, liver, egg yolks, fish, whole grains, beans and nuts.

Vitamin B6 (pyridoxine)

- helps process amino acid to make new tissue

- helps metabolize fat and carbs

- strengthens the immune system

- eliminates premenstrual fluid excess

- improves the skins appearance

- reduces muscle cramps and pains on the legs

- prevents, nausea and numbing of the hands

- keeps sodium and phosphorus levels in check

Symptoms of Vitamin B6 deficiency include: nervousness, insomnia, rashes, dermatitis, and loss of muscle control, anemia, low learning capabilities and water retention.

Foods high in vitamin B6 include: breads, cereals, grains, seeds, chicken, fish, meats and veggies.

Vitamin B12 (cobalamin)

- helps in the formation and regeneration of red cells that help prevent anemia

- is necessary to metabolize fat, carbs and protein

- keeps the nervous system healthy

- helps infants and children with their growth

- increases energy

- is needed to absorb calcium

Symptoms of vitamin B12 deficiency are: lack of appetite, high risk of getting chronic anemia, tiredness, slow growth in kids, spinal cord degeneration and depression.

Foods high in vitamin B12 include: meat, chicken, fish, milk and eggs.

Biotin:

- helps use up protein, folic acid and vitamin B12

- helps restore hair

Biotin deficiency symptoms include: extreme tiredness, dizziness, muscle pains, loss of appetite, dry, brittle hair, hair loss, depression, and dull, dry skin.

Foods high in Biotin are: peas, oatmeal, fresh soybeans, nuts, seeds, brown rice and kefir.

Folic Acid (folate) is essential for:

- transportation of the necessary coenzymes for metabolizing amino acids in the body

- for child growth

- total fetal development in pregnant women

- reproduction of new cells

Folic acid is found in sprouted wheat, fresh green leafy vegetables (especially raw spinach), beans, lettuce, carrots, tomatoes, parsley, broccoli, wheat germ, egg yolk, asparagus, lamb, liver[1]), and salmon.

Symptoms of folic acid deficiency are: gastrointestinal problems, anemia, arteriosclerosis, osteoporosis, depression, Vitamin B12 deficiency, and premature grey hair. Lack of folic acid during pregnancy can damage the fetus; the baby may be born with spinal bifida, meningocele, anencephaly.

Foods rich in folic acid, water soluble vitamins: lettuce, carrots, tomatoes, parsley, spinach, broccoli and wheat germ.

Inositol is recommended in doses of 100 to 500mg per day and forms part of the B complex and of the body tissues.

The main function of Inositol is to:

- aid the body in the manufacture of lecithin[2] which helps transport fat from the liver to cells

- assist in avoiding high cholesterol

---

1   Liver is not recommended for pregnant women due to the possibility of an overdose of Vitamin A.

2   Lecithin is naturally-produced by our bodies, but only if we eat cereals made with bran and wheat, oatmeal, eggs, fruit, cow liver, or veal, liver, and wheat germ. Lecithin is made in the liver, goes to the intestine, and is absorbed by the blood.

Lecithin is also produced naturally by our body but only if we eat food that contain lecithin: bran and wheat cereals, oatmeal, eggs, fruit, cow liver or veal and germ wheat. Lecithin is produced in the liver, goes through the intestines and absorbed by the blood.

Foods that have inositol include: brewer's yeast, fruits, beans, milk, raisins, vegetables, whole grain oats, whole grain wheat, and sprouted grains.

Inositol deficiency symptoms can be: high blood pressure, high cholesterol, constipation eczema, and hair loss.

CHOLINE is necessary to:

- control fat and cholesterol in the body

- keep fat from accumulating in the liver

- help the kidney and gallbladder

- improve the nervous system, memory, and membrane cells

Taken together, the Vitamin B complex and Vitamin C help keep the liver and the nervous system in optimum conditions, and with it the elimination of fat from the body is more complete. Part of choline is made in our organism with the help of a fatty acid known as lecithin.

Choline deficiency symptoms: cirrhosis, liver degeneration, hardening of the arteries, heart problems, high blood pressure, and hemorrhages.

PABA (paraaminobenzoic acid) is a substance that works just like a vitamin. Its benefits are:

- Rapid repair of tissue and wounds, especially when caused by the sun

- Helps keep hair and skin healthy

- In charge of skin pigmentation in order to prevent or improve vitiligo.

People who are allergic to this substance must take lecithin in order to help their bodies produce PABA.

Vitamin C is important because of how essential it is to:

- produce and strengthen collagen[3]

- promote bone growth and to heal any bone problem

- assist with iron absorption

- reduce infections and strengthen the immune system

- prevent the formation of carcinogenic cells

- get rid of free radicals that poison the blood with metals such as led, aluminum, chromium, etc...

Symptoms of Vitamin C deficiency: difficulty healing wounds, frequent or recurring colds or infections, and problems associated with the respiratory system.

---

3   Collagen connects all tissues in the body; without it, tissues cannot repair or grow.

Foods high in Vitamin C are: parsley, broccoli, bell peppers, strawberries, citrus fruits (lemons, oranges, and grapefruit), papaya, cauliflower, kale, mustard greens, cantaloupe and Brussels sprouts.

Vitamin E is a potent natural antioxidant that:

- protects cells from toxins, toxic metals, drugs, and free radicals

- helps the immune system

- improves sight

- prevents premature aging

- strengthens the nervous system

- has healing properties

- is considered to be an anti-carcinogen

Some of the symptoms of Vitamin E deficiency are: irritability, water retention, nervous system problems, fatigue, attention problems, and deficiency in the immune system.

Foods high in Vitamin E are: grape seed oil, soy oil, brown rice, multi-grain cereals, sprouted grain cereals, and green leafy vegetables.

Vitamin D is necessary for the well-being of your teeth, gums, bones, and calcium absorption.

Its deficiency causes osteoporosis at an early age, gum disease, and diseases of the skin and teeth.

Foods high in Vitamin D include: green leafy vegetables, plain yogurt, almonds, kefir, cheese, butter, oysters, and fish.

COOKING TIPS

Let your imagination go wild and cook whatever healthy food you like. Eat whatever you want, however you want, except fried foods, refined sugar, and bleached flours. Use brown rice, sprouted grain bread, tortillas, cereals, oats, rye, and bran. Use plain yogurt, kefir, whey, green salads, chicken, and fish. When my nutrition plan tells you to drink milk and eat fruit, it means you can use plain yogurt, fresh or frozen fruit to make a shake. To sweeten your shake, use bee honey or stevia. If you make a milkshake (preferably using almond milk) with a delicious apple or banana, you do not need sugar. Moderate your banana consumption to 3 times a week tops.

Here are some sample recipes to get you started:

BEEF:

Try a meatball soup with vegetables and instead of making the balls with meat and white rice use brown rice. You can also make the traditional shredded beef *picadillo* without California chilies or green tomatoes if you suffer from ulcers, gastritis, colitis, or gastrointestinal problems.

The famous *carne asada* may be served with salad and grilled vegetables or you can make guacamole with shredded meat and serve it with vegetable soup, or a grated, raw vegetable salad. You can also make beef with *adobo* and put it in the refrigerator all night so it can have a better flavor.

Another easy and delicious way of preparing beef is by mixing:

- ¼ pound of premium ground beef

- 1 raw egg

- ¼ yellow bell pepper

- 2 mushrooms

- 4 crushed garlic cloves

- ¼ of an onion

- 3 tablespoons of parsley

- 1 tablespoon of fresh oregano

- 1 tablespoon of fresh cilantro

- Sea salt to taste

All fresh vegetables and herbs must be very finely-chopped before mixing them with the meat; then you make something similar to hamburger patties only thinner and bigger, to put on a *comal*.

In a few minutes you will notice that they look ready to be turned over, so turn them over. Serve them with green salad and the famous *molcajete chile* or guacamole and steamed veggies. If you need bread or tortillas you can have 1 serving of sprouted bread or tortilla. Because they don't have gluten, your stomach can digest them more easily. You also can use big lettuce leaves like tortillas.

CHICKEN:

Make traditional *calabacitas con carne puerco* (zucchini with pork), but instead of using pork use chicken, turkey or quail. Another way you can cook chicken is making it in *adobo* and putting it in the oven with fresh herbs or in its own juices (no water added) with veggies, tomato, onions and fresh cloves of garlic.

Chicken breast fillet grilled with lemon juice, salt, pepper and some other spices such as fresh herbs like, basil, oregano, dill, rosemary, etc. is a quick and tasty dish.

More chicken—place chicken meat that has been seasoned with garlic, 1 whole onion, and 5 or 6 bay leaves and 1 cup of the following sauce (do not add water).

Blend:

- 3 boiled tomatoes

- 1 California chili

- 1 clove of raw garlic

- Sea salt to taste

Add this sauce to the chicken and cook it on a low flame. Serve with a portion of semi-raw vegetables, lettuce salad, cucumber, avocado, tomato, carrot, shredded zucchini and cabbage; as dressing use one lemon, sea salt and olive oil.

POTATOES:

Bake potatoes in the oven and serve them with clarified butter (you can find it at health food stores). Baked potatoes go well with grilled chicken or fish fillet and raw vegetables. When you eat potatoes do not eat rice, bread or tortilla for better digestion.

Another way to prepare baked potatoes is to mash them while they are still hot and add vinegar and jalapeño chilies, finely chopped celery, pickled jalapeños, grated carrots and a bit of butter (1 tablespoon per potato).

If for whatever reason you cannot eat vinegar or tolerate peppers, add skimmed milk or plain yogurt, sea salt, clarified butter, chopped garlic and pepper after mashing the potatoes.

NOTE: If you still suffer from obesity, have boiled potatoes with lemon, pepper and olive oil only once or twice per week. If you don't need to lose weight you can have them 2 or 3 times per week. Regardless, if you suffer obesity or diabetes you must eat potatoes in small portions no more than 3 times per week.

FISH:

Fish can be baked, steamed in its own juice, or grilled. The secret lies in using different kinds of condiments, spices and vegetables every time you cook it.

If you steam the fish you can add some bell peppers, onion, tomato, garlic, pepper and sea salt and serve it with asparagus and a raw salad made with mushrooms and green leaf lettuce with no dressing. Just add lemon, sea salt and olive oil.

BROWN RICE:

Because brown rice is complete, it takes longer to cook. Soak it all night ahead of time, and it will take about 45 minutes to cook. Season it with sea salt, pepper and crushed garlic. You can serve it with black beans, Greek yogurt and cucumber salad with tomatoes, marinated onion (in lemon and sea salt), finely- chopped cabbage, lemon and olive oil.

Another way to serve brown rice is to soak it for 14 hours and rinse it before cooking. Once it puffs, add soy cream to taste and 4 or 5 teaspoons of chopped almonds. You can also add a bit of manuka honey so that it gives it the delicious final touch and top it with 1 sliced boiled egg. This plate is high in proteins and will give you energy to keep burning fat. Manuka honey can be found in any health food store.

For those of you who like Mexican rice, brown rice is a good substitute. Toast the rice with or without oil. If you use oil, use grape seed oil. Then, once the rice has been toasted, add the previously-prepared tomato sauce with tomatoes, onion and a bit of fresh chopped oregano. Add chicken broth, cover it and let it simmer until the rice cooks and fluffs. Serve the dish with the following salad: use romaine leaf lettuce and add green apples and pears cut in slices; add nuts almonds or pine nuts, cranberries with no additives, lemon, olive oil, and a teaspoon of balsamic vinegar.

The fruits that you add to your salad are considered to be 1 of the 2 portions allowed for the day, so don't overdo it on sugar even if it's from natural fruit. Lastly, accompany the brown rice and salad with grilled eggplant slices seasoned with sea salt and pepper.

NOTE: Brown rice is a meat, chicken, fish, potato, and legumes substitute. If you eat brown rice do not eat bread, potatoes, or tortillas. If you wish to lose weight faster, do not eat rice with red meat; instead, eat a small portion of chicken or fish. It is best if you use brown rice for dinner only 2 or 3 times per week.

SALAD:

The following salad can be served 2 or 3 times per week; besides all the vegetables you can add the following: chicken, tuna, boiled eggs, or legumes such as string beans, garbanzos or kidney beans.

Boil potatoes, carrots, celery, peas, green beans, garbanzos or kidney beans and make sure that only the potato is well-cooked. The rest of the vegetables have to be semi-cooked in order to get the full advantage of their properties. Cut all the vegetables in small cubes and chop up a small tomato and cabbage.

Put all the vegetable together and add the fish, preferably fresh tuna (if you don't have fresh tuna use canned). You can replace tuna with boiled chicken breast previously seasoned and shredded. Mix everything and add lemon, sea salt, fresh garlic, and olive oil.

PROTEIN:

Prepare the famous skewers or bruschettas with chicken, lean beef, and fish. On each skewer put a piece of meat, then add a piece of bell pepper, 1 cherry tomato, a chunk of onion, a fish chunk, another piece of bell pepper, a tomato, the onion, and so on until the skewer is full. Season it to taste with fresh herbs, crushed garlic, and sea salt. Turn the grill or the oven on and cook. Once they are ready, brush the skewers with olive oil and lemon.

FRUITS AND VEGETABLES

FRUITS

Apples: Help stabilize blood sugar levels, lower blood pressure, soothe appetite and lower cholesterol.

Avocados: Have a great combination of essential fatty acids to help the body control cholesterol, they improve skin problems such as acne and premature wrinkles, and they regulate blood pressure and prevent constipation because they are high in fiber.

Bananas: Are good for the heart because of their high potassium content; they are good for the circulatory system and they help you sleep better.

Grapes: Have plenty of Potassium and are good for people with heart problems; they stop mucous formation in the big intestine, clean up the face, liver, intestines and kidneys.

Pears: Give a lot of energy, have a lot of fiber, and help prevent and cure constipation. Pears contain Folic Acid and Vitamin C. They also neutralize the nervous system.

Strawberries: Have plenty of Vitamin C which helps revive the immune system. Strawberries are also good for the heart, have plenty of natural fiber to cure constipation and diminish colon cancer, help nourish bones and teeth. They clean the blood system and cure depression.

Mangoes: Give a lot of energy, neutralize the nervous system, and have Vitamins A, C and Beta Carotene to attack the harmful oxygen molecules known as free radicals.
Oranges: They are good for sight, the skin, the circulatory system and the mucous membrane; they help the digestive and urinary systems, they repair tissue and strengthen the immune system.

Papaya: Has a lot of carotenoids or antioxidant pigmentation—phytochemicals essential for the heart's health and to strengthen the immune system. When they say that papaya has a lot of carotenoids it is because it has twice as many antioxidants as other fruits, which makes this fruit a healing food to help prevent all kinds of cancer. It is also a digestive agent that not only helps digest foods properly but it also cures stomach and digestive problems; it prevents ulcers and cures stomach irritations caused by excessive medications. Papaya, guavas, pineapples and other citrus fruits help make collagen to repair tissue, nerves and muscles, strengthen the immune system and act like antioxidants by protecting the Vitamins A and E from damage by toxins and chemicals and they help normalize cholesterol.

Peaches: They help keep you young and beautiful because they have 3 types of antioxidants.

Kiwi: Have plenty of antioxidants as well as Vitamin C and they help get rid of toxic radicals in the body. They also help improve the look of skin and hair.

VEGETABLES

Zucchinis: High in Vitamins A, and C, Potassium and Calcium. The best zucchinis are those that are less than 6 inches in length.

Tomatoes: Rich in Vitamins C and A, B complex, Potassium and Phosphorus; its antioxidants help prevent prostate cancer.

Asparagus: Anti-cancerous and high in glutathione that protect small veins that could break, they protect against radiation and are high in Vitamins, A, C and E, B complex, Potassium and Zinc. They are excellent at reducing inflammation of the prostate and protecting against cancer.

Avocados: Have more potassium than bananas and can be mixed with carrot juice to make dressing to put over raw vegetables and salads.

Mustard Greens: This anti-cancerous vegetable is recommended for people with autoimmune diseases, arthritis and/or depression. This is a spicy vegetable, so use it in small amounts and dilute with water.

Parsley: Excellent for the digestive system, it purifies the bloodstream, is anti-cancerous, and has more Vitamin C than oranges. Parsley also has twice as much iron as spinach, is high in Vitamin A, Magnesium and Copper, 2 minerals that cure bad breath.

Parsley Root: Eliminates water retention, regulates menstruation, and is high in Vitamin A, Niacin, Complex B, Magnesium, Iron and Potassium. It helps with urinary problems, kidney and digestive

problems as well as abdominal pain, inflammation and flatulence. The root has 3 times as much Vitamin C as the leaf.

Celery Root: High in Potassium, Vitamin C, Magnesium, Calcium, Iron, B12, B8, B5, Zinc, fiber and protein.

Onion: It detoxifies; it is anti-allergic and antiviral.

Kale: Protects from colon cancer, is high in Vitamins A and C, is a decongestant, heals the digestive system, helps the liver burn fat and improves the immune system.

Kohlrabi: Related to cabbage, it is high in fiber, Potassium, Magnesium, Vitamins A and C, Folic Acid and Calcium and is an antioxidant. It improves any health problem, helps regulate glucose and is recommended for people who have diabetes or hypoglycemia. The smaller it is the more nutrients it has. It is used in stews and in raw vegetable juices.

IMAGINE

THAT THIS IS YOUR LUNCH

AND DINNER PLATE...

DIVIDE IT INTO FOUR PARTS

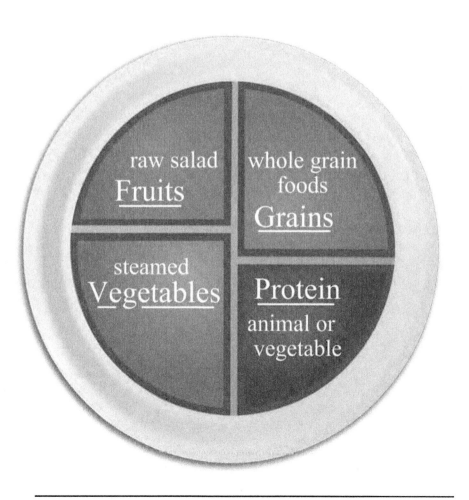

PLATE EXPLANATION

On the 1st quarter of your plate you can put 3 or 4 of the following raw vegetables (make sure you rotate them). You can also add small pieces of fruit:

- Asparagus

- Celery

- Fresh Cucumber

- Bell Peppers

- Mushrooms

- Spinach

- Red or Green Leaf Lettuce

- Butter Lettuce

- Romaine Lettuce

- Arugula

- Kale

- Oak Leaf Lettuce

- Onion

- Tomato

- Grated Carrot

- Grated Zucchini

- Jlcama

- Sunflower Seeds

- Almonds

- Dry Fruit

- Sprouted Grains or Alfalfa

On the 2nd quarter of your plate you can add 2 or 3 of the following steamed vegetables and rotate them:

- Artichokes

- Asparagus

- Cauliflower

- Cabbage

- Broccoli

- Brussels sprouts

- Beets

- Zucchini

- Eggplant

- Bell Pepper

- Mushrooms

- Turnips

- Bok Choy

- Okra

- Collard Greens

- Kale

- Mustard Greens

- Spinach

- Sweet Potato

- Hubbard Squash

On the 3rd quarter of your plate put 1 of the following proteins:

- Chicken

- Fish

- Turkey

- Lean Beef

- Veal

- Lamb

- Goat

- Green Beans

- Peas

- Lentils

- Garbanzo

- Lima Beans

- Green Beans

On the 4th quarter of your plate put 1 of the following grains (carbohydrates):

- Brown Rice

- Buck Wheat

- Quinoa

- Wild Rice

- Sprouted Grain Bread

- Sprouted Grain Tortilla

- Brown Rice Pasta (gluten free)

- Potato

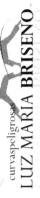

Luz María Briseño's Nutrition Guide

curvaspeligrosas
LUZ MARIA BRISEÑO

Breakfast	Breakfast	Breakfast	Breakfast	Breakfast	Breakfast	Breakfast
Vegetable Smoothie / Oatmeal / Skim Milk or Soy Milk / Fresh Fruit	Vegetable Smoothie / 2 Egg Whites / Asparagus / Bell Pepper / Tomato / Fresh Fruit	Baked Tostada / Tostada w/ Beans & Lettuce / Tomato / Milk / Fruit	Vegetable Smoothie / Cactus or Green Beans / with egg whites / Milk / Fruit	Vegetable Smoothie / 3/4 cups of "sweet potato" / Olive Oil / Nuts / Milk	Hotcakes made from oatmeal or Wheat flour / Dices Fruit / Soy Milk	Fruit / 3 Egg Whites / Soy Milk or Fat Free Milk / 3 nuts

Lunch	Lunch	Lunch	Lunch	Lunch	Lunch	Lunch
Grilled Chicken Wrap / 1 tortilla / Avocado / Lettuce / Mushrooms / Tomato / Bell Pepper / Cilantro / Jalapeño	On the Grill: / Liver or Fish / Vegetable Salad / Medium size Potato / Fruit	½ Sandwich & ½ Salad / Whole grain bread, low sodium turkey / Vegetables / Fruit	Garbanzo Bean Soup with vegetables / 1 tortilla / Fruit	Shake using Soy or Skim Milk / ½ apple or berries / Almonds / 20gm of Whey or Soy Protein	Bean salad with brown rice / vegetables (bell pepper, cucumber, mushrooms, dried tomatoes / olive oil	Vegetarian Sandwich with avocado, cucumber, alfalfa germ or lettuce, tomato, bell pepper, and a fruit salad

Dinner	Dinner	Dinner	Dinner	Dinner	Dinner	Dinner
½ Fish or Chicken Sandwich / Whole Grain Bread / Vegenaise / Fruit Salad / Almonds	½ Soup & ½ Salad with olive oil, fruits & nuts	Salad / Small portion of whole wheat pasta with mushroom & tomato sauce / Fruit	Beef or Chicken / Vegetables / Olive Oil / Salad / A slice of bread or tortilla / Fruit	Soup or Salad of legumes* / Tortilla / Fruit	Fish or Chicken / Vegetables / Olive Oil / Brown Rice Salad / Fruit	Salmon or Lentil Soup / Vegetables / Olive Oil / Salad / Fruit

Supper	Supper	Supper	Supper	Supper	Supper	Supper
½ Fish or Chicken Sandwich / Salad / Olive Oil	Chicken Soup with vegetables & brown rice (no tortilla)	Protein Vegetable Soup: Lentil, garbanzo, beans, peas, carrot, potato, celery, parsley, tomato, cilantro, onion / corn or germinated tortillas	Fish / Salad / Olive Oil / 1 Potato	Brown Rice & Beans / Avocado / Tomato Salsa / Salad with Olive Oil	Tofu or Green Beans / Cucumber Salad / Olive Oil / 1 Hard Boiled Egg or three Egg Whites	Lentil or Broad Bean Soup / Salad / Olive Oil / Vegetables

SNACK IDEAS: Eat only one a day

- Snacks between breakfast and lunch: ½ fruit & natural fat free yogurt
- Protein snack for night emergencies: 2 lettuce leafs with 2 slices of turkey ham low in sodium & 2 tomato slices
- Snack during the day: Low fat cottage cheese with fruit
- Snack during the day: ½ of an apple with 1 tablespoon of almond or peanut butter
- Snack during the day: ½ of a celery stick with almond butter
- Snack during the day: ½ cup of garbanzo soup

INSTRUCTIONS FOR A GOOD NUTRITIONAL PLAN

At the beginning of your day, the recommended vegetable juice or water with lemon, according to the breakfast ideas table, you can take 1 of the 2 that may be available to you 15 minutes prior to breakfast.

When you decide to eat an egg with ½ a cup of vegetables, I recommend grating them or chopping them finely and making and omelet with one tablespoon of grape seed oil. You can eat it with sprouted grain bread or tortilla and a cup of almond or soy milk.

Make sure you add some sort of seed to your salads and some kind of oil such as olive, grape seed, avocado or sesame instead of commercial dressings. Garnish with sea salt, pepper, fresh crushed garlic and a bit of lemon juice or apple cider vinegar.

It is preferred if the bread or tortilla you eat is made from flourless sprouted grains or 100% bran.

Oatmeal must be natural, boiled in water and sweetened with raw bee's honey or using the sweetener stevia. Milk may be of almonds or soy. Yogurt must be natural. Green vegetable smoothies of choice must be homemade (prepared by you).

The animal protein serving should be approximately the size of the palm of the person who is going to eat it and as thick as a deck of cards. No meat should be fried; everything should be steamed, baked, cooked in its own juices, in stew, grilled or with a bit of grape seed oil. Grape seed oil is for salads; not for cooking.

The vegetable portion is one cup (rotate them). The salad can be lettuce based, some days with cucumbers, shredded carrots and tomatoes other days it can be with pear, jicama, peppers, grapes, etc..., to make a rainbow of a salad. Ideal dressings are those you make with extra virgin olive oil, sea salt, fresh crushed garlic and lemon.

You must eat every 3 hours. The latest you can eat is 3 hours before bedtime. It does not matter what time you start your day, your breakfast must be eaten when you wake up even if that is 2:00 pm. It is better to drink water between meals (10 /8oz. glasses per day).

Reduce stress with physical exercise.

Exercising is vital 3 to 5 times per week in order to be healthy and stay at your ideal weight.

www.curvaspeligrosas.net

WEEKLY PROGRESS TABLE

Name: _____

Date	Weight	Size

BEFORE

PICTURE
(OPTIONAL)

AFTER

PICTURE
(OPTIONAL)

(DON'T WEIGH YOURSELF EVERY DAY)

WEEKLY PROGRESS TABLE

Name: _____

Date	Weight	Size

BEFORE

PICTURE
(OPTIONAL)

AFTER

PICTURE
(OPTIONAL)

BIOGRAPHY

I am Mexican. For over 20 years I have worked in the Spanish language radio industry in both northern and southern California.

I have been working for over 10 years as a broadcaster; my career took an unexpected turn from musical radio to talk radio. The first nutrition radio show was called *Curvas Peligrosas* (dangerous curves) and it happened without planning it. Several years ago, I was hospitalized for 4 days; 2 of them in a comma due to heart weakness (lack of potassium).

My lifestyle had been anything but healthy. I only slept 3 hours each night; I would wake up at 3:30 or 4:00 am and I started work at 5:00 am. I did not sleep during the day, or eat well. I did not like water because it made me rush to the bathroom, and truthfully, I was lazy to go. My favorite foods were coffee with bagels or donuts, and right after work I'd eat a hamburger with fries and a "diet" soda, fried chicken or fried tacos and one or two chocolate bars. In the evening my dinner was a banana split or some other dessert high in refined sugar and calories. No wonder I could not sleep.

Since I was a child I had suffered of insomnia while at the same time, sugar and synthetic foods were the base of my diet. I was always sickly during my adolescence and adult life. When I was 11 years old, I was already being prescribed medicine to help with my nervousness. While I was pregnant with my only son, Mateo, I was hospitalized 3 times due to kidney infections. After he was born, I stayed hospitalized for several months due to serious health problems. At age 25 I was diagnosed with asthma due to poorly-treated chronic allergies, lack of water and excess sugars throughout my life. I had hypothyroidism, hyperthyroidism, candidiasis, dehydration and severe depression. The last time I was hospitalized with heart problems a doctor told me, with an indifferent tone in his voice, *"Child, if you don't learn how to eat well, you are going to die."*

That is when I began to research what I should be eating. Over 10 years ago, I began studying nutrition because I needed to make some changes. Now I do it because it is my passion.

Later the same year after I had been in a comma and returned to work, I conducted a 2 week survey on what my radio listeners' New Year's resolutions were. Most of them (both men and women), wanted to lose weight and improve their health. So, I asked my radio programmer, Pepe Garza, to allow me to give nutrition tips on what I had been learning and was fascinated with, on the air. Pepe thought it was a good idea; he even helped me develop the program. And that is how the nutrition show *Curvas Peligrosas* got started. That passion for nutrition grew and it helped make me a Certified Nutritionist-Broadcaster.

My passion for nutrition has surged because nutrition saved my life. Today I thank God that I no longer use steroids to control my asthma attacks, or any other medication for thyroid or depression. My mission now is to help those who need and want to be helped through radio shows, advice on nutrition through television, internet and my nutrition seminars.

ABOUT THE AUTHOR

Luz Maria Briseño, CNC is a Spanish language radio broadcaster in northern and southern California. Her first nutrition radio show was *Curvas Peligrosas*. Her education includes Hartnell College (Salinas, CA); San Jose State (San Jose, CA); Vocalization Classes with Professor Bob Corff (Hollywood, CA) and Wellness and Nutrition AFPA USA (Ship Bottom, NJ).

Favorite pastimes for Ms. Briseño include books on nutrition, psychology, neuro-linguistics; horror, drama and animated moves; rock, jazz and romantic music, shopping and traveling.

CPSIA information can be obtained at www.ICGtesting.com
Printed in the USA
LVOW04s1120210515

439349LV00013B/71/P